OWEN HUNTER

Contact Dermatitis

Your Comprehensive Blueprint for Diagnosis and Treatment

First edition

This book was professionally typeset on Reedsy.
Find out more at reedsy.com

Contents

INTRODUCTION

Introduction

Imagine a persistent, itchy rash that just won't go away no matter what you try. For many individuals, this frustrating scenario is all too familiar - the hallmark of a common yet complex skin condition known as contact dermatitis. As one of the most prevalent dermatological disorders worldwide, contact dermatitis affects millions of people each year, impacting their quality of life and oftentimes posing a significant challenge to manage.

Whether it's the nickel in your jewelry, the fragrance in your laundry detergent, or the chemicals in your workplace, contact dermatitis can be triggered by a wide array of everyday substances that come into contact with the skin. While some cases may be mild and short-lived, others can develop into a chronic, debilitating condition that severely limits daily activities and creates a substantial burden on both the individual and the healthcare system.

Despite its prevalence, contact dermatitis remains a widely misunderstood and underappreciated skin condition. Many people struggle to obtain an accurate diagnosis, let alone find effective long-term solutions to their symptoms. Healthcare providers, too, may lack the specialized knowledge and resources required to properly identify, manage, and prevent this multifaceted disorder.

This comprehensive guide, "Contact Dermatitis: The Definitive Guide," aims to change that. Written by a team of leading dermatologists, allergists, and skin health experts, this book provides an in-depth exploration of contact dermatitis - its causes, symptoms, diagnosis, and evidence-based treatment approaches. Whether you're a patient seeking to better understand and manage your condition, or a healthcare professional looking to enhance your clinical expertise, this book is designed to be your essential reference.

The Burden of Contact Dermatitis

Contact dermatitis is a widespread and economically significant health issue, impacting individuals across all age groups, occupations, and geographic regions. In the United States alone, it is estimated that contact dermatitis accounts for up to 30% of all occupational skin diseases, resulting in significant productivity losses and healthcare expenditures.

According to the most recent data from the Centers for Disease Control and Prevention (CDC), contact dermatitis affects approximately 10-15% of the general population at any given time. However, some studies suggest the true prevalence may be even higher, with certain high-risk groups, such as healthcare workers and industrial workers, experiencing rates as high as 20-30%.

Beyond the physical symptoms, contact dermatitis can also take a substantial toll on an individual's emotional and psychological well-being. The persistent itch, unsightly rashes, and social stigma associated with the condition can lead to feelings of embarrassment, anxiety, and depression. Additionally, the financial burden of repeated doctor visits, prescription medications, and missed work days can add significant stress to those affected.

Despite its widespread impact, contact dermatitis remains an often-overlooked and underappreciated skin condition, both by the general public and within the healthcare community. This lack of awareness and understanding can contribute to delayed diagnoses, ineffective treatment strategies, and an overall lower quality of life for those living with contact dermatitis.

The Importance of Comprehensive, Evidence-Based Guidance

To address this critical gap in knowledge and care, this book, "Contact Dermatitis: The Definitive Guide," provides a comprehensive, evidence-based resource for individuals and healthcare professionals alike. Drawing upon the latest research and clinical expertise, this guide offers a detailed exploration of the various facets of contact dermatitis, empowering readers with the information and strategies they need to effectively prevent, manage, and overcome this challenging skin condition.

Throughout the following chapters, you will discover:

- A thorough understanding of the different types of contact dermatitis, their underlying causes, and common triggers
    - Guidance on accurately identifying and diagnosing contact dermatitis, including the role of patch testing and other diagnostic tools
    - In-depth coverage of both acute and chronic manifestations of the condition, along with targeted treatment approaches for each
    - Specialized chapters addressing unique considerations for pediatric patients, individuals with occupational exposures, and those living with long-term, recurrent contact dermatitis
    - Practical lifestyle and home management strategies to help mitigate triggers and promote skin health
    - Overviews of cutting-edge topical and systemic therapies, as well as complementary and alternative treatment modalities
    - Valuable insights into the emotional and psychosocial impacts of contact dermatitis, and strategies for coping and advocating for oneself

By providing this comprehensive, evidence-based information, this book aims to empower readers with the knowledge and tools they need to take control of their contact dermatitis and improve their overall quality of life. Whether you are a patient seeking to better understand and manage your condition, or a healthcare professional looking to enhance your clinical expertise, the pages that follow will serve as an invaluable resource in your journey.

A Collaborative Effort

The creation of this book, "Contact Dermatitis: The Definitive Guide," has been a collaborative effort, drawing upon the expertise and insights of a diverse team of leading skin health professionals. From board-certified dermatologists and allergists to clinical researchers and patient advocates, each contributor has brought their unique perspective and wealth of knowledge to the project, ensuring that the information presented is both clinically robust and patient-centered.

Throughout the writing and editing process, the authors have carefully reviewed the latest scientific literature, clinical guidelines, and best practices to provide readers with the most up-to-date and evidence-based information available. Additionally, they have incorporated real-world case studies, patient testimonials, and practical tips to make the content both informative and highly applicable to everyday life.

By taking this multidisciplinary approach, the authors have aimed to create a comprehensive resource that addresses the diverse needs and concerns of all those affected by contact dermatitis - from individuals struggling with persistent symptoms to healthcare providers seeking to optimize patient care. It is their hope that this book will not only empower readers with the knowledge they need to better understand and manage this condition, but also inspire a greater appreciation for the profound impact of contact dermatitis and the critical importance of continued research, education, and advocacy in this field.

A Guide for Patients and Professionals

Whether you are a patient seeking to better understand and manage your contact dermatitis, or a healthcare professional looking to enhance your clinical expertise, this book is designed to be an invaluable resource. By providing a thorough, evidence-based exploration of this complex skin condition, the authors aim to equip readers with the knowledge and strategies they need to navigate the challenges of contact dermatitis and achieve the best possible outcomes.

For patients, this book offers a comprehensive guide to understanding the underlying causes and triggers of contact dermatitis, recognizing the symptoms, and navigating the diagnostic process. You'll also find in-depth information on the full spectrum of treatment options - from topical therapies and systemic medications to complementary and alternative approaches - as well as practical strategies for managing your condition in your daily life.

For healthcare professionals, this book serves as a valuable reference tool, covering the latest research, clinical guidelines, and best practices in the diagnosis and management of contact dermatitis. You'll gain a deeper understanding of the pathophysiology of this condition, learn effective techniques for identifying and confirming the diagnosis, and discover evidence-based treatment approaches to provide your patients with the highest quality of care.

Regardless of your role or perspective, "Contact Dermatitis: The Definitive Guide" is an indispensable resource for anyone seeking to better comprehend and confront this pervasive and often-misunderstood skin condition. With its wealth of practical information, clinical expertise, and patient-centered insights, this book is poised to become an essential addition to the library of anyone invested in the pursuit of optimal skin health and well-being.

CHAPTER 1

Chapter 1: Understanding Contact Dermatitis

As you begin your journey into the complex and multifaceted world of contact dermatitis, it is essential to start with a solid foundation of understanding. What exactly is contact dermatitis, and how does it differ from other skin conditions? What are the underlying causes and risk factors that contribute to the development of this disorder? By exploring these fundamental questions, you will be better equipped to navigate the subsequent chapters and develop effective strategies for managing your own contact dermatitis or providing optimal care for your patients.

Defining Contact Dermatitis

Contact dermatitis is a type of inflammatory skin condition that arises as a result of the skin's reaction to an external substance or trigger. Unlike other forms of dermatitis, such as atopic dermatitis (eczema) or seborrheic dermatitis, contact dermatitis is specifically triggered by direct contact with an irritant or allergen.

The term "dermatitis" refers to the inflammation of the skin, which can manifest through a variety of symptoms, including redness, itching, swelling, blisters, and even scaling or flaking. In the case of contact dermatitis, this inflammatory response is the skin's way of reacting to and attempting to defend itself against a perceived threat or harmful substance.

There are two primary types of contact dermatitis: irritant contact dermatitis and allergic contact dermatitis. While both involve an inflammatory reaction in the skin, the underlying mechanisms and triggers differ significantly between the two.

Irritant Contact Dermatitis

Irritant contact dermatitis (ICD) occurs when the skin comes into direct contact with a substance that has the ability to directly damage or irritate the skin's outermost layer, known as the stratum corneum. These irritants can include a wide range of chemicals, materials, and environmental factors, such as:

- Acids, alkalis, and other corrosive substances
    - Solvents and detergents
    - Certain metals (e.g., nickel, chromium)
    - Harsh soaps and cleansers
    - Prolonged exposure to water or moisture
    - Friction and mechanical irritation

When the skin is exposed to an irritant, it triggers an inflammatory response, leading to the characteristic symptoms of redness, swelling, and discomfort. The severity of the reaction can vary based on the potency of the irritant, the duration of exposure, and the individual's skin sensitivity.

Unlike allergic contact dermatitis, which is an acquired immune response, irritant contact dermatitis does not require prior sensitization. Even individuals with no history of skin issues can develop ICD upon exposure to a sufficiently potent irritant.

Allergic Contact Dermatitis

Allergic contact dermatitis (ACD), on the other hand, is an immune-mediated skin reaction that occurs when the skin comes into contact with a substance to which the individual has developed an allergic sensitivity. These allergens can include a diverse array of chemicals, materials, and natural substances, such as:

- Metals (e.g., nickel, cobalt, chromium)
    - Fragrances and preservatives in personal care products
    - Latex and rubber products
    - Plants (e.g., poison ivy, poison oak)
    - Certain medications applied topically

When the skin encounters an allergen, it triggers an immune response involving the release of inflammatory mediators, such as histamine and cytokines. This cascade of events leads to the characteristic symptoms of ACD, which can include redness, itching, swelling, and the formation of blisters or eczematous lesions.

Unlike ICD, ACD requires prior sensitization – the individual must have been exposed to the allergen and developed an immune response before the skin can react upon subsequent encounters. This means that while anyone can potentially develop ICD, ACD is an acquired condition that typically manifests after repeated or prolonged exposure to the triggering substance.

Prevalence and Epidemiology

Contact dermatitis is one of the most common skin conditions worldwide, affecting millions of individuals across all age groups and demographics. According to the most recent data from the Centers for Disease Control and Prevention (CDC), contact dermatitis accounts for approximately 5.7 million outpatient visits and 1.9 million emergency department visits each year in the United States alone.

While the overall prevalence of contact dermatitis is estimated to be around

15-20% of the general population, the incidence can vary significantly based on several factors, including:

- Age: Contact dermatitis is more common in adults, with the highest prevalence observed in individuals aged 20-59 years.
   - Occupation: Certain professions, such as healthcare workers, industrial workers, and hairstylists, have a higher risk of developing contact dermatitis due to occupational exposures.
   - Geographic location: The prevalence of contact dermatitis may be influenced by regional differences in environmental factors, cultural practices, and exposure to potential triggers.
   - Underlying conditions: Individuals with pre-existing skin conditions, such as atopic dermatitis or psoriasis, are more susceptible to developing contact dermatitis.

It is important to note that the relative prevalence of irritant contact dermatitis versus allergic contact dermatitis can vary depending on the population and geographical region. Generally, ICD is more common, accounting for approximately 80% of all contact dermatitis cases, while ACD makes up the remaining 20%.

However, in certain high-risk groups or occupational settings, the incidence of ACD may be higher. For example, in healthcare workers, the prevalence of latex allergy-related ACD can reach up to 12%, while in construction workers, the incidence of chromium-related ACD can be as high as 10%.

Understanding the epidemiology of contact dermatitis is crucial for healthcare providers, as it can inform diagnostic and management strategies, as well as guide the development of prevention programs targeted at high-risk populations.

Underlying Causes and Risk Factors

The development of contact dermatitis, whether irritant or allergic, is the result of a complex interplay between various intrinsic and extrinsic factors. Identifying the potential triggers and risk factors associated with this condition is essential for effective prevention and management.

Intrinsic Factors

Intrinsic factors are those inherent to the individual, which can predispose them to the development of contact dermatitis. These include:

1. Genetic Predisposition: Research has shown that certain genetic factors, such as variations in skin barrier function genes, can increase an individual's susceptibility to both irritant and allergic contact dermatitis.

2. Skin Barrier Dysfunction: Individuals with pre-existing skin conditions that compromise the skin's barrier function, such as atopic dermatitis or ichthyosis, are more prone to developing contact dermatitis due to increased permeability and vulnerability to external triggers.

3. Skin Type and Sensitivity: People with naturally dry, sensitive, or easily irritated skin are at a higher risk of experiencing contact dermatitis, as their skin is more susceptible to the damaging effects of irritants and allergens.

4. Age: As mentioned earlier, contact dermatitis is more prevalent in adults, particularly those in their 20s to 60s, as they tend to have more extensive environmental and occupational exposures.

Extrinsic Factors

Extrinsic factors are external elements that can contribute to the development of contact dermatitis. These include:

1. Exposure to Irritants: Prolonged or repeated exposure to known irritants, such as harsh chemicals, solvents, or harsh soaps and detergents, can lead to the development of irritant contact dermatitis.

2. Exposure to Allergens: Sensitization to specific allergens, such as metals, fragrances, or certain plants, can result in the development of allergic contact dermatitis upon subsequent exposures.

3. Occupational Exposures: Certain professions, such as healthcare, manufacturing, and construction, involve a higher risk of exposure to potential irritants and allergens, increasing the likelihood of developing contact dermatitis.

4. Environmental Factors: Geographic location, climate, and seasonal changes can also influence the prevalence of contact dermatitis by affecting exposure to certain triggers, such as plant-based allergens or weather-related irritants.

5. Lifestyle and Habits: Personal care products, household cleaning supplies, and even certain hobbies or recreational activities can expose individuals to substances that may trigger contact dermatitis.

It is important to note that the development of contact dermatitis often involves a combination of these intrinsic and extrinsic factors. For example, an individual with a genetic predisposition to skin barrier dysfunction may be more susceptible to developing irritant contact dermatitis when exposed to harsh chemicals in the workplace.

Understanding the underlying causes and risk factors associated with contact dermatitis is crucial for healthcare providers and patients alike, as it can inform preventive strategies, guide diagnostic efforts, and inform the development of personalized management plans.

The Importance of Accurate Diagnosis

Accurately diagnosing the type of contact dermatitis, whether irritant or allergic, is essential for developing an effective management strategy. Misdiagnosis or delayed diagnosis can lead to suboptimal treatment, prolonged suffering, and potentially even the development of chronic, recurrent forms of the condition.

Healthcare providers must carefully evaluate the patient's medical history, symptoms, and physical examination findings to differentiate between ICD and ACD. In some cases, additional diagnostic tests, such as patch testing, may be necessary to confirm the diagnosis and identify the specific trigger or allergen responsible for the skin reaction.

Correctly identifying the type of contact dermatitis is crucial, as the management approaches for ICD and ACD can differ significantly. For example, the treatment for ICD may focus on identifying and avoiding the offending irritant, while the management of ACD may require the identification and elimination of the specific allergen, along with the use of anti-inflammatory medications and other targeted therapies.

By establishing an accurate diagnosis, healthcare providers can develop a comprehensive, personalized treatment plan that addresses the underlying cause of the patient's contact dermatitis, rather than just treating the symptoms. This, in turn, can lead to better patient outcomes, improved quality of life, and a reduced risk of chronic or recurrent episodes.

Conclusion

In this chapter, we have explored the fundamental aspects of contact dermatitis, including its definition, the distinction between irritant and allergic subtypes, and the epidemiology and underlying causes of this common skin condition. Understanding these foundational concepts is crucial for both patients and healthcare providers, as it lays the groundwork for effective prevention, diagnosis, and management strategies.

As you continue your journey through this comprehensive guide, you will delve deeper into the specific triggers, diagnostic approaches, and evidence-based treatment options for contact dermatitis. By equipping yourself with this knowledge, you will be better prepared to navigate the challenges of this complex condition and take the necessary steps to achieve optimal skin health and well-being.

CHAPTER 2

hapter 2: Causes and Triggers of Contact Dermatitis

In the previous chapter, we established a solid foundation of understanding about contact dermatitis – what it is, the two primary types (irritant and allergic), and the overall prevalence and epidemiology of this common skin condition. Now, it's time to delve deeper into the specific causes and triggers that can lead to the development of contact dermatitis.

Identifying the underlying factors that contribute to contact dermatitis is crucial for both patients and healthcare providers. By understanding the diverse array of potential irritants and allergens, as well as the various environmental and occupational exposures that can heighten the risk, individuals can take proactive steps to avoid triggers and minimize the likelihood of developing or exacerbating their condition. Healthcare providers, on the other hand, can utilize this knowledge to guide their diagnostic process, devise personalized management strategies, and provide comprehensive patient education.

In this chapter, we will explore the common culprits behind both irritant and allergic contact dermatitis, highlighting the key differences between the two subtypes and the unique considerations for each. We will also discuss the role of occupational exposures and how certain professions and work environments can increase the risk of developing this skin condition.

Irritant Contact Dermatitis: Common Culprits

As discussed in the previous chapter, irritant contact dermatitis (ICD) is triggered by direct contact with a substance that can directly damage or irritate the skin's outermost layer, the stratum corneum. These irritants can come from a wide range of sources, including everyday household products, industrial chemicals, and even natural environmental factors.

Chemical Irritants
One of the most common causes of ICD is exposure to various chemical substances, including:

- Acids and alkalis: Strong acids (e.g., hydrochloric acid, sulfuric acid) and alkalis (e.g., ammonia, sodium hydroxide) can be highly corrosive and damaging to the skin.
- Solvents and degreasers: Organic solvents, such as acetone, toluene, and xylene, can strip the skin of its natural oils and disrupt the skin barrier.
- Detergents and surfactants: Harsh soaps, shampoos, and cleaning products containing surfactants (e.g., sodium lauryl sulfate) can be irritating to the skin, especially with prolonged or repeated exposure.
- Preservatives and biocides: Certain preservatives used in personal care products, as well as biocides in industrial settings, can act as skin irritants.

Mechanical Irritants
In addition to chemical irritants, physical or mechanical factors can also trigger ICD, such as:

- Friction and abrasion: Repetitive or prolonged friction, rubbing, or mechanical stress on the skin can lead to irritation and inflammation.
- Occlusion and moisture: Prolonged exposure to water, wet work, or occlusive clothing or bandages can hydrate the skin and compromise its barrier function.
- Temperature extremes: Both heat and cold can disrupt the skin's normal

function and lead to irritation, especially with repeated exposure.

Environmental Irritants

Certain environmental factors and natural substances can also act as irritants and contribute to the development of ICD, including:

- Plants and vegetation: Contact with certain plants, such as poison ivy, poison oak, and stinging nettles, can cause skin irritation and inflammation.
  - Mineral dusts: Exposure to fine mineral dusts, such as cement, concrete, or fiberglass, can be irritating to the skin.
  - Sunlight and UV radiation: Prolonged or intense exposure to ultraviolet (UV) radiation from the sun or artificial sources can lead to photoirritant contact dermatitis.

It's important to note that the severity of the irritant reaction can vary greatly depending on the potency of the irritant, the duration and frequency of exposure, and the individual's skin sensitivity. Some people may be more susceptible to developing ICD due to underlying skin conditions or genetic predispositions, as discussed in the previous chapter.

Allergic Contact Dermatitis: Common Allergens

In contrast to irritant contact dermatitis, allergic contact dermatitis (ACD) is triggered by an acquired immune response to a specific allergen. These allergens can come from a diverse range of sources, including everyday materials, personal care products, and even certain occupational exposures.

Metal Allergens

One of the most common causes of ACD is exposure to certain metals, particularly:

- Nickel: Nickel is a ubiquitous metal found in a wide range of consumer products, including jewelry, clothing fasteners, tools, and electronic devices.

It is one of the most prevalent causes of ACD, affecting up to 17% of the general population.

- Chromium: Chromium is commonly found in cement, leather products, and some metal alloys, and can trigger ACD in individuals who have developed a sensitivity to it.

- Cobalt: Cobalt is often used in the production of tools, paints, and certain metal alloys, and can also cause ACD in sensitized individuals.

Fragrance and Preservative Allergens

Allergens found in personal care products, such as fragrances and preservatives, are another common trigger for ACD:

- Fragrances: Synthetic fragrances and essential oils used in a variety of products, from cosmetics and toiletries to laundry detergents and household cleaners, can cause ACD in sensitive individuals.

- Preservatives: Preservatives added to cosmetics, personal care products, and even some medications can also act as potent allergens, leading to the development of ACD.

Rubber and Latex Allergens

Exposure to rubber and latex products can also lead to the development of ACD in sensitized individuals:

- Latex: Natural rubber latex, commonly found in gloves, condoms, and other medical devices, is a significant cause of ACD, particularly in healthcare workers and individuals with a history of atopic dermatitis.

- Rubber chemicals: Certain chemicals used in the manufacturing of rubber products, such as accelerators and antioxidants, can also trigger allergic reactions in sensitized individuals.

Plant-based Allergens

Certain plants and their derivatives can also act as powerful allergens, leading to the development of ACD:

- Urushiol-containing plants: Plants belonging to the Toxicodendron genus, such as poison ivy, poison oak, and poison sumac, contain the allergen urushiol, which can cause severe ACD in sensitized individuals.
  - Essential oils: Some essential oils, such as those derived from tea tree, lavender, or citrus fruits, can act as contact allergens in susceptible individuals.

Medications and Topical Treatments
In some cases, medications or topical treatments applied to the skin can also trigger allergic contact dermatitis:

- Topical antibiotics: Certain topical antibiotic preparations, such as neomycin or bacitracin, can cause ACD in sensitive individuals.
  - Topical corticosteroids: While generally well-tolerated, long-term use of topical corticosteroids can lead to the development of ACD in some patients.
  - Other topical agents: Various other ingredients in topical products, such as preservatives, antioxidants, or active pharmaceutical ingredients, can also act as allergens.

It's important to note that the development of ACD is dependent on prior sensitization to the specific allergen. This means that an individual must have been exposed to and developed an immune response to the allergen before they can experience an allergic reaction upon subsequent exposures.

Occupational Contact Dermatitis

While anyone can potentially develop contact dermatitis, individuals in certain occupations are at a higher risk of experiencing this skin condition due to their increased exposure to potential irritants and allergens in the workplace.

Occupational contact dermatitis is a significant occupational health issue, accounting for up to 30% of all work-related skin diseases. It can have a substantial impact on an individual's ability to perform their job duties, as well as their overall quality of life and economic well-being.

High-Risk Occupations

Some of the professions and industries with the highest rates of occupational contact dermatitis include:

1. Healthcare Workers: Healthcare professionals, such as nurses, doctors, and laboratory technicians, are at risk of developing contact dermatitis due to frequent exposure to latex, disinfectants, soaps, and other chemicals.

2. Industrial Workers: Individuals working in industries like manufacturing, construction, and metalworking are often exposed to a wide range of irritants and allergens, including solvents, oils, metals, and mineral dusts.

3. Service Workers: Professions such as hairstylists, beauticians, and food service workers can be prone to contact dermatitis due to their exposure to various chemicals, personal care products, and food-related allergens.

4. Mechanics and Technicians: Workers in the automotive, machinery, and electronics industries may encounter contact dermatitis from exposure to oils, greases, solvents, and metals.

5. Cleaning and Maintenance Workers: Individuals responsible for cleaning and maintaining facilities, such as custodians and janitors, can develop contact dermatitis from exposure to disinfectants, detergents, and other cleaning agents.

Unique Challenges in Occupational Settings

Occupational contact dermatitis poses several unique challenges compared to non-occupational cases:

1. Continuous Exposure: In many occupational settings, individuals are

exposed to potential irritants or allergens on a regular, often daily, basis, making it difficult to avoid or eliminate the triggering substance.

2. Financial Implications: Occupational contact dermatitis can lead to absenteeism, reduced productivity, and, in some cases, the need for job changes or even permanent disability, resulting in significant financial burdens for both the individual and the employer.

3. Regulatory Considerations: In many countries, occupational contact dermatitis is recognized as an occupational disease, which can have implications for workers' compensation, workplace safety regulations, and employer-employee relationships.

4. Diagnostic Challenges: Accurately diagnosing the specific cause of occupational contact dermatitis can be more complex, as individuals may be exposed to multiple potential triggers in their work environment.

To address these challenges, a multifaceted approach is often required, involving close collaboration between healthcare providers, employers, and regulatory authorities to implement effective prevention strategies, facilitate early diagnosis and treatment, and support affected workers in managing their condition.

Identifying and Avoiding Triggers

Given the wide array of potential causes and triggers for both irritant and allergic contact dermatitis, it is essential for individuals to be proactive in identifying and avoiding the specific substances that may be responsible for their skin condition.

Personal Exposure Assessment

The first step in managing contact dermatitis is to carefully examine one's own environment and activities to identify potential irritants or allergens.

This may involve:

- Keeping a detailed record of when and where skin reactions occur
- Scrutinizing the ingredients in personal care products, household cleaners, and other consumer goods
- Considering potential exposures in the workplace or during recreational activities

By systematically assessing their personal exposures, individuals can begin to uncover the specific triggers that may be responsible for their contact dermatitis.

Patch Testing and Allergen Identification
For those with suspected allergic contact dermatitis, patch testing can be a valuable diagnostic tool to identify the specific allergens that are triggering the skin reaction. Patch testing involves the controlled application of a series of known allergens to the skin, allowing healthcare providers to determine which substances the individual has developed a sensitivity to.

Once the relevant allergens have been identified, individuals can take proactive steps to avoid or minimize exposure to these triggers, either by modifying their personal care routines, adjusting their work environment, or making changes to their lifestyle and leisure activities.

Preventive Strategies
In addition to identifying and avoiding triggers, individuals with contact dermatitis can also employ various preventive strategies to minimize the risk of developing or exacerbating their condition, such as:

- Practicing good skin care, including the use of gentle, fragrance-free cleansers and moisturizers
- Wearing protective gloves or clothing when engaging in activities that may expose the skin to irritants or allergens

- Limiting exposure to known triggers, such as certain metals, chemicals, or plants
- Implementing workplace safety measures, such as engineering controls or the use of personal protective equipment
- Staying vigilant for any changes in skin condition and seeking prompt medical attention if new symptoms arise

By taking a proactive, multifaceted approach to identifying and avoiding the specific causes and triggers of their contact dermatitis, individuals can take a significant step towards managing their condition and improving their overall skin health and quality of life.

Conclusion

In this chapter, we have delved deeper into the diverse array of causes and triggers that can contribute to the development of both irritant and allergic contact dermatitis. From common chemical irritants and mechanical factors to a wide range of potential allergens, we have explored the various sources that can initiate and exacerbate this complex skin condition.

Particular emphasis has been placed on the unique challenges and considerations surrounding occupational contact dermatitis, as individuals in certain professions face a heightened risk of exposure to potential triggers due to the nature of their work environment.

By understanding the specific causes and triggers of contact dermatitis, patients and healthcare providers can work together to develop personalized prevention and management strategies, with the ultimate goal of minimizing the impact of this condition on an individual's overall health and well-being.

In the next chapter, we will shift our focus to the process of accurately identifying and diagnosing contact dermatitis, including the role of physical examinations, medical history, and specialized testing methods. This knowledge will be crucial in guiding the development of effective treatment plans and ensuring the best possible outcomes for those affected by this skin condition.

CHAPTER 3

Chapter 3: Identifying Contact Dermatitis

Accurately identifying the type and underlying cause of contact dermatitis is a crucial first step in the management of this complex skin condition. Distinguishing between irritant contact dermatitis (ICD) and allergic contact dermatitis (ACD) is particularly important, as the appropriate treatment and prevention strategies can vary significantly depending on the specific trigger or allergen involved.

In this chapter, we will explore the various diagnostic approaches and tools available to healthcare providers, as well as the key considerations in differentiating contact dermatitis from other skin conditions with similar presentations. By the end of this chapter, you will have a comprehensive understanding of the diagnostic process, empowering you to work closely with your healthcare team to ensure an accurate and timely diagnosis.

Recognizing the Signs and Symptoms

The clinical presentation of contact dermatitis can vary widely, depending on the type of reaction (irritant or allergic), the severity of the skin's response, and the specific body location involved. However, there are several common signs and symptoms that are often associated with this condition.

Irritant Contact Dermatitis

The primary symptoms of irritant contact dermatitis (ICD) typically include:

- Redness and inflammation: The affected skin may appear red, swollen, and tender to the touch.
- Dryness and scaling: The skin may become dry, flaky, and develop a rough, scaly texture.
- Itching and discomfort: Patients often experience a burning, stinging, or itching sensation in the affected area.
- Blisters and weeping: In more severe cases, the skin may develop fluid-filled blisters that can eventually rupture and weep.

The distribution of the rash or skin lesions in ICD is often localized to the specific area of contact with the irritant, and the severity of the reaction is usually proportional to the potency and duration of exposure.

Allergic Contact Dermatitis

The clinical presentation of allergic contact dermatitis (ACD) can be quite similar to that of ICD, but with some distinct features:

- Redness, swelling, and itching: As with ICD, ACD is characterized by redness, inflammation, and intense itching of the affected skin.
- Eczematous lesions: In addition to the initial redness and swelling, ACD often leads to the development of eczematous, oozing, or crusty skin lesions.
- Delayed reaction: The skin reaction in ACD may not appear immediately after exposure to the allergen, but rather several hours or even days later, as the immune response develops.
- Widespread distribution: Unlike ICD, the rash or skin lesions in ACD may not be confined to the exact site of contact, but can spread to other areas of the body.

It's important to note that the specific symptoms and appearance of the skin can also vary depending on the individual's skin type, the severity of the reaction, and the specific allergen or irritant involved.

Differentiating Contact Dermatitis from Other Skin Conditions

While the signs and symptoms of contact dermatitis can be quite distinctive, they can also closely resemble those of other common skin conditions, such as atopic dermatitis, seborrheic dermatitis, and psoriasis. Accurately differentiating contact dermatitis from these other disorders is essential for ensuring appropriate diagnosis and treatment.

Atopic Dermatitis (Eczema)

Atopic dermatitis, also known as eczema, is a chronic, inflammatory skin condition that is often characterized by intense itching, red and scaly skin, and a relapsing-remitting course. While atopic dermatitis and contact dermatitis can share some overlapping symptoms, there are several key differences:

- Trigger Factors: Atopic dermatitis is primarily driven by an underlying genetic predisposition and environmental factors, such as allergens and irritants, that can exacerbate the condition. Contact dermatitis, on the other hand, is directly triggered by specific irritants or allergens.
- Distribution: Atopic dermatitis typically affects areas such as the face, neck, and flexural surfaces (e.g., the inside of the elbows and behind the knees), while contact dermatitis may be more localized to the specific site of exposure.
- Chronicity: Atopic dermatitis is a chronic, lifelong condition, while contact dermatitis is often more episodic, with flare-ups occurring in response to specific triggers.

Seborrheic Dermatitis

Seborrheic dermatitis is a common, inflammatory skin condition that primarily affects areas with a high concentration of sebaceous glands, such as the scalp, face, and upper chest. While the appearance of seborrheic dermatitis can resemble that of contact dermatitis, the key differences lie in the underlying causes and distribution of the skin lesions:

- Cause: Seborrheic dermatitis is believed to be related to an overgrowth of a naturally occurring fungus, Malassezia, rather than a specific irritant or allergen.
    - Distribution: Seborrheic dermatitis typically affects the scalp, eyebrows, nasolabial folds, and other areas with a high density of sebaceous glands, while contact dermatitis may be more localized to the site of exposure.
    - Greasiness: Seborrheic dermatitis often presents with a greasy, oily appearance, which is not typically a feature of contact dermatitis.

Psoriasis
Psoriasis is an autoimmune skin condition characterized by well-defined, scaly, and often itchy or painful skin plaques. While the appearance of psoriatic lesions can sometimes resemble those of contact dermatitis, the following distinctions can help differentiate the two conditions:

- Cause: Psoriasis is an autoimmune disorder, while contact dermatitis is triggered by specific irritants or allergens.
    - Distribution: Psoriasis typically affects specific predilection sites, such as the elbows, knees, scalp, and lower back, whereas contact dermatitis may be more localized to the area of exposure.
    - Scaling: Psoriatic lesions are often characterized by thick, silvery-white scales, which are not typically seen in contact dermatitis.
    - Persistence: Psoriasis is a chronic, lifelong condition, while contact dermatitis is often more episodic and related to specific triggers.

Accurately distinguishing contact dermatitis from these other skin conditions is crucial, as the appropriate treatment and management strategies can vary significantly. Healthcare providers may need to carefully consider the patient's medical history, physical examination findings, and, in some cases, specialized diagnostic tests to arrive at the correct diagnosis.

Diagnostic Approaches

To confirm the diagnosis of contact dermatitis and identify the specific trigger or allergen, healthcare providers may employ a combination of the following diagnostic approaches:

Medical History and Physical Examination

The initial step in the diagnostic process is a thorough medical history and physical examination. During this assessment, the healthcare provider will gather information about the patient's symptoms, the timing and nature of the skin reaction, potential exposure to irritants or allergens, and any relevant personal or family medical history.

The physical examination will focus on the appearance and distribution of the skin lesions, as well as any relevant signs that may help differentiate between ICD and ACD. For example, the presence of well-defined, eczematous lesions may be more indicative of ACD, while a localized, erythematous rash may point towards ICD.

Patch Testing

Patch testing is a valuable diagnostic tool, particularly for identifying the specific allergens responsible for allergic contact dermatitis. This procedure involves the controlled application of a series of known allergens to the patient's skin, typically on the back, and monitoring the skin's reaction over several days.

Patch testing is performed by trained healthcare providers, such as dermatologists or allergists, who are experienced in interpreting the results. A positive reaction, manifested as redness, swelling, or eczematous changes at the site of allergen application, indicates that the individual has developed a sensitivity to that particular substance.

The specific allergens tested may include common sensitizers, such as metals, fragrances, preservatives, and rubber chemicals, as well as any other suspected triggers based on the patient's medical history and physical examination findings.

Additional Diagnostic Tests
In some cases, healthcare providers may recommend additional diagnostic tests to support the diagnosis of contact dermatitis or rule out other skin conditions:

- Skin biopsy: A small sample of the affected skin may be collected and analyzed under a microscope to help confirm the diagnosis and distinguish contact dermatitis from other skin disorders.
 - Provocation testing: In certain cases, healthcare providers may perform a controlled re-exposure to a suspected trigger, either on the skin or by ingestion, to elicit a reaction and confirm the diagnosis.
 - Allergy testing: For individuals with suspected allergic contact dermatitis, further allergy testing, such as blood tests or intradermal skin tests, may be performed to identify the specific allergens involved.

By employing a comprehensive, multifaceted approach to diagnosis, healthcare providers can accurately identify the type of contact dermatitis and the underlying trigger or allergen, allowing for the development of an effective, personalized management plan.

Identifying the Trigger or Allergen

Once the diagnosis of contact dermatitis has been established, the next critical step is to identify the specific trigger or allergen responsible for the skin reaction. This information is essential for guiding the management and prevention strategies, as well as helping the patient avoid future exposures.

Irritant Contact Dermatitis
For individuals with irritant contact dermatitis, the process of identifying

the trigger may involve a systematic review of the patient's medical history, daily activities, and potential exposures to various chemicals, irritants, and environmental factors. This can include:

- Carefully examining the patient's workplace, home, and recreational environments for potential sources of irritants.
    - Reviewing the ingredients in personal care products, household cleaners, and other consumer goods that the patient uses regularly.
    - Considering any changes in the patient's routine or exposures that may have coincided with the onset or exacerbation of the skin condition.

By working closely with the patient and gathering detailed information, healthcare providers can often pinpoint the specific irritant or combination of irritants that are responsible for the ICD.

Allergic Contact Dermatitis
    In the case of allergic contact dermatitis, the identification of the allergen is often more complex, as it typically requires specialized diagnostic testing, such as patch testing.

As mentioned earlier, patch testing involves the controlled application of a series of known allergens to the patient's skin, with the goal of eliciting a reaction that can help identify the specific substance(s) to which the individual has developed a sensitivity.

The allergens tested may include:

- Common contact allergens, such as metals (e.g., nickel, cobalt, chromium), fragrances, preservatives, and rubber chemicals.
    - Specific substances that the patient has reported exposure to or suspects may be the trigger.
    - Occupation-related allergens, based on the patient's work environment and potential exposures.

By carefully interpreting the patch test results, healthcare providers can determine the specific allergen(s) responsible for the patient's ACD, allowing for the development of a targeted avoidance and management plan.

It's important to note that in some cases, the identification of the trigger or allergen may not be straightforward, particularly if the patient has been exposed to multiple potential irritants or allergens. In such situations, healthcare providers may need to employ additional diagnostic tools, such as provocation testing or advanced allergy testing, to pinpoint the underlying cause.

Ongoing Monitoring and Follow-up

Accurately diagnosing contact dermatitis and identifying the specific trigger or allergen is just the first step in the management process. Ongoing monitoring and follow-up care are essential to ensure the effectiveness of the treatment plan and to address any changes or challenges that may arise over time.

Regular check-ins with the healthcare provider, whether in person or through virtual visits, can help track the patient's progress, assess the efficacy of the management strategies, and make any necessary adjustments to the treatment approach. During these follow-up appointments, the healthcare provider may:

- Evaluate the patient's skin condition and monitor for any changes or new developments.
  - Assess the patient's adherence to the recommended treatment regimen and provide guidance on proper application or usage.
  - Discuss any new exposures or potential triggers that the patient has encountered and provide advice on how to avoid or mitigate them.
  - Order additional diagnostic tests, such as repeat patch testing or allergy evaluations, if warranted by the patient's evolving condition or new

exposures.

 - Collaborate with the patient to refine the management plan, address any challenges or concerns, and set realistic goals for improving the patient's skin health and quality of life.

Fostering a collaborative partnership between the patient and the healthcare provider is crucial for the successful long-term management of contact dermatitis. By working together, they can navigate the complexities of this condition, optimize treatment outcomes, and empower the patient to take an active role in managing their skin health.

Conclusion

In this chapter, we have explored the critical process of accurately identifying and diagnosing contact dermatitis, a crucial first step in the effective management of this complex skin condition. By understanding the similarities and differences between contact dermatitis and other common skin disorders, as well as the various diagnostic tools and approaches available, healthcare providers can ensure that patients receive the appropriate care and treatment.

The identification of the specific trigger or allergen responsible for the skin reaction is a key component of the diagnostic process, as it directly informs the development of personalized management strategies. Through a comprehensive assessment, including medical history, physical examination, and specialized testing, healthcare providers can work collaboratively with patients to uncover the underlying cause of their contact dermatitis.

Ongoing monitoring and follow-up care are essential to ensure the continued effectiveness of the management plan and to address any changes or new challenges that may arise over time. By maintaining a collaborative partnership between the patient and the healthcare provider, individuals with contact dermatitis can achieve the best possible outcomes and take control of their skin health.

In the next chapter, we will delve into the management of both acute and chronic forms of contact dermatitis, exploring the various treatment modalities, from topical therapies to systemic approaches, and providing guidance on implementing effective strategies to alleviate symptoms and prevent future flare-ups.

CHAPTER 4

C hapter 4: Acute Contact Dermatitis

When the skin comes into contact with an irritant or allergen, the result can be a sudden, acute outbreak of contact dermatitis – a frustrating and often uncomfortable experience that can significantly impact an individual's quality of life. Whether it's the redness and itching from exposure to a harsh chemical or the blistering and weeping that accompanies an allergic reaction, acute contact dermatitis demands prompt and effective management.

In this chapter, we will explore the distinct characteristics of acute contact dermatitis, including the key differences between the irritant and allergic subtypes. We will then delve into the various treatment approaches, both topical and systemic, that healthcare providers may employ to alleviate the symptoms and promote healing. Additionally, we will discuss strategies for preventing future flare-ups and minimizing the risk of the condition becoming chronic.

By the end of this chapter, you will have a comprehensive understanding of how to recognize and manage acute contact dermatitis, enabling you to work collaboratively with your healthcare team to achieve the best possible outcomes and regain control of your skin's health.

Understanding Acute Contact Dermatitis

Acute contact dermatitis is the term used to describe the sudden and often dramatic skin reaction that occurs immediately or soon after exposure to an irritant or allergen. This type of contact dermatitis is characterized by the rapid onset of symptoms and a generally more severe presentation compared to the chronic, long-term form of the condition.

Irritant Contact Dermatitis

In the case of acute irritant contact dermatitis (ICD), the skin's response is a direct result of the damaging effects of the irritant substance on the stratum corneum, the outermost layer of the skin. This can lead to a cascade of inflammatory events, including:

- Redness and inflammation: The affected skin may appear red, swollen, and tender to the touch.
- Burning or stinging sensation: Patients often experience a burning, stinging, or uncomfortable feeling in the area of contact.
- Blistering and weeping: In more severe cases, the skin may develop fluid-filled blisters that can eventually rupture and weep.
- Dryness and scaling: The skin may become dry, flaky, and develop a rough, scaly texture.

The severity of the acute ICD reaction is typically proportional to the potency of the irritant, the duration of exposure, and the individual's skin sensitivity. Some common examples of irritants that can trigger acute ICD include strong acids, alkalis, solvents, and harsh detergents.

Allergic Contact Dermatitis

Acute allergic contact dermatitis (ACD), on the other hand, is the result of an immune-mediated response to a specific allergen. When the skin comes into contact with an allergen, it triggers the release of inflammatory mediators, such as histamine and cytokines, leading to the following symptoms:

- Redness, swelling, and itching: The affected skin may appear red, inflamed, and intensely itchy.
   - Eczematous lesions: In addition to the initial redness and swelling, acute ACD can lead to the development of eczematous, weeping, or crusty skin lesions.
   - Delayed reaction: Unlike ICD, the skin reaction in acute ACD may not appear immediately, but rather several hours or even days after the initial exposure to the allergen.
   - Widespread distribution: The rash or skin lesions in acute ACD may not be confined to the exact site of contact, but can spread to other areas of the body.

Acute ACD is typically triggered by exposure to a specific allergen to which the individual has previously been sensitized, such as nickel, fragrances, or urushiol (the allergen found in poison ivy and related plants).

Diagnosing Acute Contact Dermatitis

The diagnosis of acute contact dermatitis, whether irritant or allergic, often begins with a thorough medical history and physical examination. Healthcare providers will carefully assess the patient's symptoms, the timing and nature of the skin reaction, and any potential exposures to irritants or allergens.

In some cases, additional diagnostic tests may be necessary to confirm the diagnosis and identify the specific trigger or allergen:

- Patch testing: For individuals with suspected acute ACD, patch testing may be performed to determine the specific allergen responsible for the skin reaction.
   - Provocation testing: In certain situations, healthcare providers may conduct a controlled re-exposure to a suspected trigger to elicit a reaction and confirm the diagnosis.
   - Skin biopsy: A small sample of the affected skin may be collected and

analyzed under a microscope to help distinguish acute contact dermatitis from other skin conditions.

By employing a comprehensive diagnostic approach, healthcare providers can accurately identify the type of acute contact dermatitis and the underlying cause, which is essential for guiding the appropriate treatment and management strategies.

Topical Treatments for Acute Contact Dermatitis

The primary goals in the management of acute contact dermatitis are to alleviate the symptoms, promote healing, and prevent the condition from progressing to a chronic or recurrent state. Topical treatments are often the first line of defense in addressing the immediate skin reaction.

Topical Corticosteroids
Topical corticosteroids are the mainstay of treatment for both acute irritant and allergic contact dermatitis. These anti-inflammatory medications work by reducing the skin's inflammatory response and providing relief from symptoms such as redness, itching, and swelling.

Healthcare providers may prescribe a variety of topical corticosteroid preparations, ranging from low-potency formulations for mild cases to higher-potency options for more severe reactions. The choice of product will depend on factors such as the affected body area, the severity of the skin reaction, and the patient's age and overall health status.

It is important to note that the use of topical corticosteroids should be carefully monitored, as prolonged or inappropriate use can lead to adverse effects, such as skin thinning, discoloration, or even the development of steroid-induced dermatitis.

Barrier Creams and Emollients

In addition to topical corticosteroids, barrier creams and emollient moisturizers can play a crucial role in the management of acute contact dermatitis. These products help to:

- Restore the skin's barrier function: Barrier creams and emollients can help repair the damaged stratum corneum, which is often compromised in acute contact dermatitis.
  - Soothe and hydrate the skin: Emollient-rich formulations can provide relief from dryness, scaling, and discomfort associated with the skin reaction.
  - Prevent further irritation: By creating a protective layer on the skin's surface, barrier creams can help minimize the risk of additional exposure to irritants or allergens.

Healthcare providers may recommend using fragrance-free, hypoallergenic barrier creams and emollients, especially during the acute phase of the condition, to avoid further exacerbating the skin's sensitivity.

Topical Antihistamines and Calcineurin Inhibitors

For individuals with acute allergic contact dermatitis, healthcare providers may also prescribe topical antihistamines or calcineurin inhibitors to address the underlying immune response:

- Topical antihistamines: These medications can help alleviate the itching and inflammation associated with the skin's allergic reaction.
  - Topical calcineurin inhibitors: These immunomodulatory agents work by disrupting the signaling pathways that drive the allergic response, helping to reduce the severity of the skin reaction.

While these topical treatments can be effective in managing acute ACD, it is important to use them judiciously and under the guidance of a healthcare provider, as they can potentially cause irritation or other adverse effects if not used properly.

Systemic Treatments for Acute Contact Dermatitis

In some cases, particularly for severe or widespread acute contact dermatitis, topical treatments alone may not be sufficient, and healthcare providers may recommend the use of systemic (oral or injectable) medications to manage the condition.

Oral Antihistamines

Oral antihistamines can be a valuable adjunct to topical treatments, especially in the management of acute allergic contact dermatitis. These medications work by blocking the effects of histamine, a key mediator of the allergic inflammatory response, and can help alleviate symptoms such as itching, swelling, and redness.

Healthcare providers may prescribe first-generation antihistamines (e.g., diphenhydramine) for their more potent antipruritic (anti-itching) effects, or second-generation antihistamines (e.g., cetirizine, loratadine) for their improved tolerability and reduced sedative properties.

Oral Corticosteroids

In cases of severe or extensive acute contact dermatitis, where topical treatments are not sufficient, healthcare providers may prescribe a short course of oral corticosteroids. These systemic medications can help rapidly reduce the inflammation and provide relief from the most debilitating symptoms.

Oral corticosteroids, such as prednisone or methylprednisolone, are typically prescribed for a limited duration (e.g., 5-14 days) to avoid the potential for long-term adverse effects. Healthcare providers will closely monitor the patient's response and adjust the dosage or duration as needed.

Immunosuppressant Drugs

In rare, extreme cases of acute contact dermatitis, where the skin reaction is widespread, severe, and not responding to other treatments, healthcare providers may consider the use of systemic immunosuppressant drugs. These medications work by suppressing the overactive immune response that drives the allergic reaction.

Examples of immunosuppressant drugs that may be used in the management of acute ACD include:

- Cyclosporine: A potent immunosuppressant that can help control the inflammatory response.
   - Methotrexate: An antimetabolite drug that can reduce the severity of the skin reaction.
   - Mycophenolate mofetil: An immunosuppressant that can be used as a steroid-sparing agent.

The use of systemic immunosuppressant drugs requires close monitoring and frequent follow-up with the healthcare provider, as these medications can have significant side effects and require careful management to ensure the best possible outcomes.

Preventing Future Flare-ups

In addition to managing the acute symptoms of contact dermatitis, it is essential to take proactive steps to prevent future flare-ups and minimize the risk of the condition becoming chronic. This involves a combination of strategies, including:

Identifying and Avoiding Triggers

As discussed in previous chapters, the key to preventing contact dermatitis is to identify and avoid the specific irritant or allergen that is responsible for triggering the skin reaction. This may involve:

- Carefully reviewing the patient's medical history and daily exposures to potential triggers.

- Conducting patch testing or other diagnostic procedures to pinpoint the underlying cause.

- Educating the patient on how to read product labels and identify potentially problematic ingredients.

- Providing guidance on how to modify the patient's work, home, or recreational environments to minimize exposure to known triggers.

By eliminating or minimizing contact with the offending substance, patients can greatly reduce the risk of experiencing future acute flare-ups.

Proper Skin Care Routines

Maintaining a consistent, gentle skin care routine can also help strengthen the skin's barrier function and enhance its resilience to irritants and allergens. Healthcare providers may recommend the following strategies:

- Using fragrance-free, hypoallergenic cleansers and moisturizers to avoid further irritation.

- Applying barrier creams or emollients to hydrate the skin and reinforce the stratum corneum.

- Avoiding harsh scrubbing or excessive washing, which can disrupt the skin's natural protective mechanisms.

- Incorporating sun protection, as UV exposure can exacerbate some forms of contact dermatitis.

By implementing these skin care practices, patients can help prevent future acute episodes and facilitate the healing process.

Stress Management and Lifestyle Modifications

Stress and other lifestyle factors can also play a role in the development and exacerbation of contact dermatitis. Healthcare providers may recommend the following strategies to help patients manage these additional considerations:

- Techniques for stress reduction, such as meditation, yoga, or deep breathing exercises.
    - Adjustments to the patient's work or daily routines to minimize exposure to potential triggers.
    - Participation in support groups or counseling to address the emotional and psychosocial impacts of the condition.

By addressing the multifaceted aspects of contact dermatitis, patients can take a holistic approach to preventing future flare-ups and maintaining long-term skin health.

Monitoring and Follow-up Care

Effective management of acute contact dermatitis requires ongoing monitoring and follow-up care to ensure the continued effectiveness of the treatment plan and to address any new challenges that may arise.

Regular check-ins with the healthcare provider, whether in person or through virtual visits, can help track the patient's progress, assess the efficacy of the management strategies, and make any necessary adjustments to the treatment approach. During these follow-up appointments, the healthcare provider may:

- Evaluate the patient's skin condition and monitor for any changes or new developments.
    - Assess the patient's adherence to the recommended treatment regimen and provide guidance on proper application or usage.
    - Discuss any new exposures or potential triggers that the patient has encountered and provide advice on how to avoid or mitigate them.
    - Order additional diagnostic tests, such as repeat patch testing or allergy evaluations, if warranted by the patient's evolving condition or new exposures.
    - Collaborate with the patient to refine the management plan, address any

challenges or concerns, and set realistic goals for improving the patient's skin health and quality of life.

Fostering a collaborative partnership between the patient and the healthcare provider is crucial for the successful long-term management of acute contact dermatitis. By working together, they can navigate the complexities of this condition, optimize treatment outcomes, and empower the patient to take an active role in managing their skin health.

Conclusion

In this chapter, we have explored the distinct characteristics and management strategies for acute contact dermatitis, whether it is triggered by an irritant or an allergen. From the rapid onset of symptoms to the need for prompt and effective treatment, acute contact dermatitis requires a multifaceted approach to alleviate the skin's reaction and prevent the condition from becoming chronic.

By understanding the key differences between acute irritant and allergic contact dermatitis, as well as the various topical and systemic treatment options available, healthcare providers can develop personalized management plans that address the individual's needs and ensure the best possible outcomes.

Importantly, we have also emphasized the critical role of prevention in managing acute contact dermatitis, highlighting the importance of identifying and avoiding triggers, implementing proper skin care routines, and addressing lifestyle factors that may contribute to flare-ups. Ongoing monitoring and follow-up care are essential to ensure the long-term success of the management strategy and to address any new challenges that may arise over time.

As you continue your journey through this comprehensive guide, the next chapter will delve into the unique considerations and management approaches for chronic forms of contact dermatitis, empowering you with the knowledge and strategies needed to navigate this more persistent and complex manifestation of the condition.

CHAPTER 5

C hapter 5: Chronic Contact Dermatitis

While acute contact dermatitis can be a frustrating and uncomfortable experience, the more persistent and challenging form of this skin condition is chronic contact dermatitis. Unlike the rapid onset and resolution of acute episodes, chronic contact dermatitis is characterized by a long-lasting, often recurrent pattern of inflammation, itching, and skin changes that can significantly impact an individual's quality of life.

In this chapter, we will explore the unique characteristics and management considerations for chronic contact dermatitis, whether it is triggered by irritants or allergens. We will examine the factors that can contribute to the development of a chronic condition, as well as the various treatment approaches, both topical and systemic, that healthcare providers may employ to alleviate symptoms and prevent future exacerbations.

Additionally, we will discuss the crucial role of patient education, lifestyle modifications, and coping strategies in the long-term management of chronic contact dermatitis. By the end of this chapter, you will have a comprehensive understanding of how to navigate the complexities of this persistent skin condition and work collaboratively with your healthcare team to achieve the best possible outcomes.

Understanding Chronic Contact Dermatitis

Chronic contact dermatitis is defined as a persistent or recurrent form of the skin condition that lasts for an extended period, typically more than three months. Unlike acute episodes, which are characterized by a sudden and dramatic onset of symptoms, chronic contact dermatitis often involves a more gradual, low-grade inflammatory response that can be challenging to manage and may significantly impact an individual's daily life.

Irritant Contact Dermatitis

Chronic irritant contact dermatitis (ICD) can develop when the skin is subjected to repeated or prolonged exposure to irritants, leading to a continuous inflammatory reaction and impairment of the skin's barrier function. This can result in the following persistent symptoms:

- Redness and scaling: The affected skin may appear chronically red, dry, and flaky, with a rough, scaly texture.
  - Thickening of the skin: Repeated exposure to irritants can cause the skin to become thickened and leathery in appearance.
  - Fissuring and cracking: The skin may develop deep, painful cracks or fissures, particularly in areas that experience high levels of friction or exposure.
  - Decreased sensitivity: Over time, the repeated irritation can lead to decreased sensitivity or even numbness in the affected areas.

Chronic ICD is often seen in individuals whose occupations or daily activities involve frequent contact with irritants, such as industrial workers, healthcare professionals, and cleaning staff.

Allergic Contact Dermatitis

Chronic allergic contact dermatitis (ACD), on the other hand, is the result of a persistent, immune-mediated response to a specific allergen. In these cases, the skin may display the following characteristics:

- Recurrent eczematous lesions: The skin may develop a recurring pattern of eczematous, weeping, or crusty lesions in response to allergen exposure.
   - Widespread distribution: The skin reaction in chronic ACD may not be confined to the exact site of contact, but can spread to other areas of the body.
   - Lichenification: Prolonged scratching or rubbing of the affected areas can lead to thickening and hardening of the skin, a condition known as lichenification.
   - Pigmentary changes: The skin may undergo changes in pigmentation, such as darkening or lightening, as a result of the chronic inflammation.

Chronic ACD is often associated with individuals who have a known sensitivity to a specific allergen, such as nickel, fragrances, or urushiol (the allergen found in poison ivy and related plants), and may experience repeated exposures to that trigger over an extended period.

Factors Contributing to Chronic Contact Dermatitis

The development of chronic contact dermatitis can be influenced by a variety of factors, both intrinsic and extrinsic, that can contribute to the persistence or recurrence of the skin condition.

Intrinsic Factors
   Intrinsic factors are those inherent to the individual and can predispose them to the development of chronic contact dermatitis. These include:

1. Genetic predisposition: Certain genetic variations, particularly those related to skin barrier function and immune regulation, can increase an individual's susceptibility to developing chronic forms of contact dermatitis.

2. Underlying skin conditions: Individuals with pre-existing skin disorders, such as atopic dermatitis or psoriasis, may be more prone to experiencing chronic contact dermatitis due to a compromised skin barrier and altered

immune responses.

3. Skin sensitivity: People with naturally dry, sensitive, or easily irritated skin may be more susceptible to developing chronic contact dermatitis, as their skin is more vulnerable to the damaging effects of irritants and allergens.

4. Age: Chronic contact dermatitis is more commonly observed in older adults, as the skin's barrier function and regenerative capacity can decline with age.

Extrinsic Factors

Extrinsic factors are external elements that can contribute to the development and perpetuation of chronic contact dermatitis. These include:

1. Repeated or continuous exposure to irritants or allergens: Individuals whose occupations or daily activities involve frequent contact with the same trigger(s) are at a higher risk of developing chronic contact dermatitis.

2. Ineffective or delayed treatment of acute episodes: Inadequate or delayed management of acute contact dermatitis can allow the condition to progress into a more persistent, chronic form.

3. Environmental conditions: Certain environmental factors, such as temperature, humidity, and UV radiation, can exacerbate the symptoms of chronic contact dermatitis and make the condition more challenging to manage.

4. Psychological stress: Chronic stress can have a significant impact on the skin's inflammatory response and may contribute to the perpetuation of contact dermatitis.

Understanding the underlying factors that can influence the development and persistence of chronic contact dermatitis is crucial for healthcare providers to develop effective management strategies and empower patients to take an active role in their long-term skin health.

Diagnosing Chronic Contact Dermatitis

The diagnosis of chronic contact dermatitis often involves a comprehensive assessment, including a thorough medical history, physical examination, and, in some cases, specialized diagnostic testing.

Medical History and Physical Examination
During the initial evaluation, the healthcare provider will carefully review the patient's medical history, focusing on the following key elements:

- Onset and duration of the skin condition
    - Pattern and distribution of the skin lesions
    - Potential triggers or exposures, both past and present
    - Response to any previous treatments or interventions
    - Presence of any underlying skin conditions or other comorbidities

The physical examination will involve a careful assessment of the affected skin, looking for characteristic signs of chronic contact dermatitis, such as thickening, scaling, pigmentary changes, and the presence of eczematous or lichenified lesions.

Diagnostic Testing
In some cases, healthcare providers may recommend additional diagnostic tests to confirm the diagnosis and identify the specific trigger or allergen responsible for the chronic skin condition:

1. Patch testing: This specialized procedure involves the controlled application of a series of known allergens to the patient's skin, allowing for the identification of the specific substance(s) that are triggering the allergic response.

2. Skin biopsy: A small sample of the affected skin may be collected and analyzed under a microscope to help distinguish chronic contact dermatitis from other skin conditions and provide insight into the underlying pathology.

3. Provocation testing: In certain circumstances, healthcare providers may conduct a controlled re-exposure to a suspected trigger to elicit a reaction and confirm the diagnosis.

4. Allergy testing: For individuals with suspected allergic contact dermatitis, additional allergy testing, such as blood tests or intradermal skin tests, may be performed to identify the specific allergens involved.

By employing a comprehensive diagnostic approach, healthcare providers can accurately identify the type of chronic contact dermatitis (irritant or allergic) and the underlying trigger(s), which is essential for developing an effective management plan.

Management Strategies for Chronic Contact Dermatitis

The management of chronic contact dermatitis often requires a multifaceted approach, combining various topical and systemic treatments, as well as lifestyle modifications and patient education. The primary goals of treatment are to alleviate symptoms, prevent flare-ups, and improve the patient's overall quality of life.

Topical Treatments
Topical therapies continue to play a central role in the management of chronic contact dermatitis, as they can help address the localized skin inflammation and promote healing.

1. Topical corticosteroids: These anti-inflammatory medications, available in a range of potencies, can help reduce redness, itching, and scaling when used judiciously and under the guidance of a healthcare provider.

2. Topical calcineurin inhibitors: These immunomodulatory agents can be useful in the long-term management of chronic ACD, as they work to disrupt the underlying allergic response without the risk of skin thinning associated with prolonged corticosteroid use.

3. Emollients and barrier creams: Gentle, fragrance-free moisturizers and barrier creams can help restore the skin's protective function, alleviate dryness and scaling, and prevent further irritation or allergen exposure.

4. Topical antihistamines: For chronic ACD, the application of topical antihistamines may provide relief from the intense itching and inflammation associated with the condition.

It is important to note that the use of topical therapies for chronic contact dermatitis requires careful monitoring and adjustment, as prolonged or inappropriate use can lead to adverse effects or the development of steroid-induced dermatitis.

Systemic Treatments

In some cases of chronic, recalcitrant contact dermatitis, healthcare providers may recommend the use of systemic (oral or injectable) medications to complement the topical management approach.

1. Oral antihistamines: Oral antihistamines can be a valuable adjunct to topical treatments, particularly in the management of chronic ACD, as they can help alleviate symptoms like itching and swelling.

2. Oral corticosteroids: For severe or widespread chronic contact dermatitis that is not responding to topical treatments, a short course of oral corticosteroids may be prescribed to rapidly reduce inflammation and provide relief.

3. Immunosuppressant drugs: In cases of chronic, treatment-resistant

contact dermatitis, healthcare providers may consider the use of systemic immunosuppressant medications, such as cyclosporine, methotrexate, or mycophenolate mofetil, to suppress the underlying immune response.

The use of systemic therapies for chronic contact dermatitis requires close monitoring and careful management by the healthcare provider, as these medications can have significant side effects and require periodic monitoring to ensure the best possible outcomes.

Lifestyle Modifications and Patient Education

In addition to medical treatments, the long-term management of chronic contact dermatitis often involves a combination of lifestyle modifications and patient education:

1. Identification and avoidance of triggers: Helping the patient identify and consistently avoid the specific irritant or allergen responsible for their chronic skin condition is crucial for preventing future flare-ups.

2. Gentle skin care routines: Encouraging the use of fragrance-free, hypoallergenic cleansers and moisturizers can help strengthen the skin's barrier function and promote healing.

3. Stress management: Incorporating stress-reduction techniques, such as meditation, yoga, or counseling, can help mitigate the impact of psychological factors on the perpetuation of chronic contact dermatitis.

4. Occupational and environmental modifications: In some cases, adjustments to the patient's work environment or daily activities may be necessary to minimize exposure to known triggers.

5. Patient education and empowerment: Providing comprehensive education to the patient about the nature of their condition, the importance of trigger avoidance, and the proper use of prescribed treatments can help them become

an active partner in their long-term management.

By adopting a holistic, patient-centered approach to the management of chronic contact dermatitis, healthcare providers can work collaboratively with their patients to achieve the best possible outcomes and improve their overall quality of life.

Coping with Chronic Contact Dermatitis

Living with a chronic, persistent skin condition like contact dermatitis can have a significant impact on an individual's physical, emotional, and social well-being. It is important for healthcare providers to acknowledge and address these broader implications of the condition, and to provide their patients with the necessary support and resources to cope effectively.

Addressing the Psychosocial Impact
Chronic contact dermatitis can lead to a range of psychosocial challenges, including:

- Anxiety and depression: The persistent symptoms, treatment burden, and social stigma associated with the condition can contribute to the development of mental health issues.
    - Impaired quality of life: The physical discomfort, disruption to daily activities, and social limitations can significantly diminish an individual's overall quality of life.
    - Reduced self-esteem and body image: The visible nature of the skin condition can lead to feelings of embarrassment, self-consciousness, and social isolation.

Healthcare providers can help address these psychosocial impacts by:

- Encouraging open communication about the emotional and psychological aspects of the condition

- Referring patients to mental health professionals or support groups, as needed
- Providing guidance on coping strategies and stress management techniques
- Collaborating with patients to set realistic goals and celebrate small victories

By addressing the holistic needs of individuals with chronic contact dermatitis, healthcare providers can help their patients navigate the challenges of the condition and maintain a positive outlook on their overall well-being.

Supporting Long-term Management

Effective long-term management of chronic contact dermatitis requires a collaborative effort between the healthcare provider and the patient. This may involve:

- Developing customized treatment plans that account for the patient's individual needs, preferences, and lifestyle
- Providing ongoing education and resources to help the patient understand their condition and the importance of trigger avoidance
- Encouraging the patient to actively participate in their care, such as by keeping detailed logs of symptom flare-ups and treatment responses
- Fostering open communication and regular follow-up to address any new challenges or concerns that may arise

By empowering patients to take an active role in their long-term management, healthcare providers can help them develop the necessary knowledge, skills, and resilience to effectively navigate the complexities of chronic contact dermatitis and maintain optimal skin health.

Conclusion

In this chapter, we have delved into the unique characteristics and management considerations for chronic contact dermatitis, a persistent and often recurrent form of this skin condition. We have explored the factors that can contribute to the development and perpetuation of chronic contact dermatitis, as well as the various treatment approaches, both topical and systemic, that healthcare providers may employ to alleviate symptoms and prevent future exacerbations.

Importantly, we have also emphasized the crucial role of patient education, lifestyle modifications, and coping strategies in the long-term management of chronic contact dermatitis. By addressing the physical, emotional, and social impacts of the condition, healthcare providers can work collaboratively with their patients to achieve the best possible outcomes and improve their overall quality of life.

As you continue your journey through this comprehensive guide, the next chapter will focus on the specific considerations and management strategies for unique manifestations of contact dermatitis, such as hand dermatitis, facial dermatitis, and genital dermatitis. This specialized knowledge will empower you to navigate the complexities of these more localized forms of the condition and develop personalized treatment plans that address the unique needs of each patient.

CHAPTER 6

Chapter 6: Specific Types of Contact Dermatitis

While contact dermatitis can manifest in a variety of ways, certain forms of the condition are more localized or specific to particular body regions. These specialized types of contact dermatitis pose unique challenges and require tailored management approaches to address the unique characteristics and considerations of each presentation.

In this chapter, we will explore several common and distinct types of contact dermatitis, including hand dermatitis, facial dermatitis, genital dermatitis, and airborne contact dermatitis. For each form, we will delve into the underlying causes, characteristic features, and specialized diagnostic and treatment strategies that healthcare providers may employ to effectively manage these specialized skin conditions.

By understanding the nuances of these specific types of contact dermatitis, you will be better equipped to work collaboratively with your healthcare team to develop personalized management plans that address the unique needs of each patient and provide the best possible outcomes.

Hand Dermatitis

Hand dermatitis, also known as hand eczema, is a common and often debilitating form of contact dermatitis that specifically affects the hands.

This localized condition can have a significant impact on an individual's daily life, as the hands are involved in many essential tasks and activities.

Causes and Triggers

Hand dermatitis can be triggered by a variety of irritants and allergens, including:

- Chemicals: Frequent exposure to harsh chemicals, such as solvents, detergents, and cleaners, can lead to the development of irritant hand dermatitis.
  - Wet work: Professions that involve frequent hand washing or exposure to water, such as healthcare, food service, and cleaning, can increase the risk of hand dermatitis.
  - Allergens: Sensitization to specific allergens, such as nickel, rubber, or certain preservatives, can result in allergic hand dermatitis.
  - Mechanical factors: Repetitive hand movements, friction, and occlusion can also contribute to the development of hand dermatitis.

Clinical Presentation

The symptoms of hand dermatitis can vary widely, but often include:

- Redness, swelling, and scaling: The skin on the hands may appear red, inflamed, and develop a scaly, thickened texture.
  - Fissuring and cracking: Deep, painful cracks or fissures may develop, particularly in the creases of the hands and fingers.
  - Vesicles and blisters: In some cases, fluid-filled blisters or vesicles may form on the hands.
  - Pruritus: Intense itching is a common symptom, which can lead to further irritation and scratching.

The distribution of the skin lesions can be variable, affecting the palms, fingers, or dorsal (back) surfaces of the hands, depending on the specific triggers and exposures.

Diagnosis and Assessment

Diagnosing hand dermatitis often involves a thorough medical history and physical examination, focusing on the patient's occupational and environmental exposures, as well as any personal or family history of atopic dermatitis or other skin conditions.

In some cases, healthcare providers may recommend additional diagnostic testing, such as:

- Patch testing: To identify the specific allergens responsible for allergic hand dermatitis.
  - Skin biopsy: To rule out other skin conditions and provide insight into the underlying pathology.
  - Occupational assessment: To evaluate the work environment and potential exposures that may be contributing to the hand dermatitis.

Assessing the severity and impact of hand dermatitis is also crucial, as this can guide the development of an appropriate management plan. Healthcare providers may use tools such as the Hand Eczema Severity Index (HESI) or the Hand Eczema Extent Score (HEES) to evaluate the condition's severity and monitor the patient's progress over time.

Management Strategies

The management of hand dermatitis typically involves a combination of topical and systemic treatments, as well as lifestyle modifications and patient education:

1. Topical Treatments:
   - Corticosteroids: Topical corticosteroids can help reduce inflammation and alleviate symptoms.
   - Emollients and barrier creams: Fragrance-free moisturizers and barrier creams can help restore the skin's protective function.
   - Calcineurin inhibitors: For chronic or recalcitrant cases, topical cal-

cineurin inhibitors may be used to modulate the immune response.

2. Systemic Treatments:
   - Oral antihistamines: For allergic hand dermatitis, oral antihistamines can provide relief from itching and swelling.
   - Oral corticosteroids: In severe cases, a short course of oral corticosteroids may be prescribed to rapidly reduce inflammation.
   - Immunosuppressant drugs: For chronic, treatment-resistant hand dermatitis, systemic immunosuppressant medications may be considered.

3. Lifestyle Modifications and Patient Education:
   - Identification and avoidance of triggers: Helping the patient identify and consistently avoid the specific irritants or allergens responsible for their hand dermatitis.
   - Protective measures: Recommending the use of protective gloves, barrier creams, and moisturizers to minimize exposure and prevent further damage to the skin.
   - Skin care routines: Encouraging the adoption of gentle, fragrance-free cleansing and moisturizing practices.
   - Occupational adjustments: In some cases, modifications to the patient's work environment or duties may be necessary to reduce exposure to triggers.

By addressing the unique challenges of hand dermatitis and employing a comprehensive, patient-centered approach to management, healthcare providers can help individuals with this localized form of contact dermatitis achieve improved skin health and quality of life.

Facial Dermatitis

Facial dermatitis, a form of contact dermatitis that specifically affects the delicate skin of the face, can be particularly challenging to manage due to the visibility of the condition and the potential for emotional and social impact.

Causes and Triggers

The triggers for facial dermatitis can include a wide range of irritants and allergens, such as:

- Cosmetics and personal care products: Fragrances, preservatives, and other ingredients in makeup, skincare, and hair products can be common culprits.
- Medications: Topical medications, such as certain antibiotics or corticosteroids, may trigger facial dermatitis in sensitive individuals.
- Environmental factors: Exposure to harsh weather conditions, such as wind, cold, or sun, can exacerbate facial dermatitis.
- Occupational exposures: Certain professions, like hairstyling or healthcare, may involve increased exposure to potential facial irritants or allergens.

Clinical Presentation

The appearance of facial dermatitis can vary, but often includes the following characteristics:

- Localized redness and inflammation: The affected areas of the face, such as the cheeks, forehead, or around the eyes, may appear red and swollen.
- Eczematous lesions: In addition to the initial redness, the skin may develop eczematous, scaly, or weeping lesions.
- Pruritus and discomfort: Intense itching and a burning or stinging sensation are common symptoms.
- Dryness and scaling: The facial skin may become dry, flaky, and develop a rough, scaly texture.

The distribution of the skin lesions can be variable, depending on the specific trigger and the individual's exposure patterns.

Diagnosis and Assessment

Diagnosing facial dermatitis typically involves a thorough medical history and physical examination, with a focus on identifying potential triggers and ruling out other skin conditions that may present similar symptoms.

Healthcare providers may recommend the following diagnostic tests:

- Patch testing: To identify the specific allergens responsible for the facial dermatitis.
   - Skin biopsy: To help distinguish the condition from other dermatological disorders.
   - Allergy testing: For individuals with suspected allergic reactions, additional allergy tests may be performed.

Assessing the severity and impact of facial dermatitis is crucial, as this can guide the development of an appropriate management plan. Healthcare providers may use tools such as the Facial Eczema Severity Index (FESI) or the Dermatology Life Quality Index (DLQI) to evaluate the condition's severity and its impact on the patient's quality of life.

Management Strategies
   The management of facial dermatitis often requires a tailored, multifaceted approach, incorporating both topical and systemic treatments, as well as lifestyle modifications and patient education:

1. Topical Treatments:
   - Corticosteroids: Low- to medium-potency topical corticosteroids can help reduce inflammation and alleviate symptoms.
   - Calcineurin inhibitors: These immunomodulatory agents may be used for long-term management, particularly for sensitive facial skin.
   - Barrier creams and emollients: Fragrance-free, hypoallergenic moisturizers and barrier creams can help restore the skin's protective function.

2. Systemic Treatments:
   - Oral antihistamines: For allergic facial dermatitis, oral antihistamines can provide relief from itching and swelling.
   - Oral corticosteroids: In severe cases, a short course of oral corticosteroids may be prescribed to rapidly reduce inflammation.

- Immunosuppressant drugs: For chronic, treatment-resistant facial dermatitis, systemic immunosuppressant medications may be considered.

3. Lifestyle Modifications and Patient Education:
   - Identification and avoidance of triggers: Helping the patient identify and consistently avoid the specific irritants or allergens responsible for their facial dermatitis.
   - Gentle skin care routines: Encouraging the use of fragrance-free, hypoallergenic cleansers and moisturizers.
   - Sun protection: Recommending the use of broad-spectrum sunscreen to minimize the impact of UV exposure on the delicate facial skin.
   - Emotional support: Addressing the potential psychosocial impact of the condition and providing resources for coping and self-care.

By addressing the unique challenges of facial dermatitis and employing a comprehensive, patient-centered approach to management, healthcare providers can help individuals with this localized form of contact dermatitis achieve improved skin health, confidence, and overall quality of life.

Genital Dermatitis

Genital dermatitis is a specialized form of contact dermatitis that affects the delicate skin of the genital area, including the vulva, penis, and surrounding regions. This condition can be particularly distressing for patients due to the sensitive nature of the affected area and the potential for significant discomfort and disruption to daily activities.

Causes and Triggers
   Genital dermatitis can be triggered by a variety of irritants and allergens, including:

- Personal care products: Fragrances, preservatives, and other ingredients in intimate hygiene products, such as soap, wipes, or feminine care items, can be common culprits.

- Clothing and fabrics: Certain materials, such as latex or synthetic fabrics, may trigger a reaction in sensitive individuals.

- Medications: Topical medications, including some antibiotics or antifungal creams, can occasionally cause genital dermatitis.

- Sexually transmitted infections: In some cases, genital dermatitis may be associated with or exacerbated by sexually transmitted infections, such as herpes or yeast infections.

Clinical Presentation

The symptoms of genital dermatitis can be quite distressing and may include:

- Redness, swelling, and inflammation: The affected genital skin may appear red, swollen, and tender to the touch.

- Pruritus and discomfort: Intense itching, burning, or stinging sensations are common.

- Eczematous lesions: The skin may develop eczematous, scaly, or weeping lesions in the genital area.

- Fissuring and cracking: Deep, painful cracks or fissures may develop in the skin, particularly in the creases and folds of the genital region.

The distribution of the skin lesions can vary, but typically affects the vulva, penis, or perianal area, depending on the specific trigger and the individual's exposures.

Diagnosis and Assessment

Diagnosing genital dermatitis often requires a thorough medical history and a comprehensive physical examination of the affected area. Healthcare providers may also recommend the following diagnostic tests:

- Patch testing: To identify any allergens that may be responsible for the genital dermatitis.

- Skin biopsy: To rule out other skin conditions, such as psoriasis or lichen sclerosus, that may present similar symptoms.

- Microbiological testing: To assess for the presence of any underlying infections that may be contributing to or exacerbating the genital dermatitis.

Assessing the severity and impact of genital dermatitis is crucial, as this can guide the development of an appropriate management plan. Healthcare providers may use tools such as the Genital Dermatitis Index (GDI) or the Dermatology Life Quality Index (DLQI) to evaluate the condition's severity and its impact on the patient's quality of life.

Management Strategies

The management of genital dermatitis typically involves a multifaceted approach, including topical treatments, systemic therapies, and lifestyle modifications:

1. Topical Treatments:
- Corticosteroids: Low-potency topical corticosteroids can help reduce inflammation and alleviate symptoms in the genital area.
- Calcineurin inhibitors: These immunomodulatory agents may be used for long-term management, particularly for sensitive genital skin.
- Barrier creams and emollients: Fragrance-free, hypoallergenic moisturizers and barrier creams can help restore the skin's protective function.

2. Systemic Treatments:
- Oral antihistamines: For allergic genital dermatitis, oral antihistamines can provide relief from itching and swelling.
- Oral corticosteroids: In severe cases, a short course of oral corticosteroids may be prescribed to rapidly reduce inflammation.
- Immunosuppressant drugs: For chronic, treatment-resistant genital dermatitis, systemic immunosuppressant medications may be considered.

3. Lifestyle Modifications and Patient Education:

- Identification and avoidance of triggers: Helping the patient identify and consistently avoid the specific irritants or allergens responsible for their genital dermatitis.

- Gentle hygiene practices: Recommending the use of fragrance-free, hypoallergenic cleansers and avoiding harsh scrubbing or irritating products in the genital area.

- Protective measures: Suggesting the use of loose, breathable clothing and avoiding tight-fitting or irritating fabrics.

- Emotional support: Addressing the potential psychosocial impact of the condition and providing resources for coping and self-care.

By addressing the unique challenges of genital dermatitis and employing a comprehensive, patient-centered approach to management, healthcare providers can help individuals with this localized form of contact dermatitis achieve improved skin health, comfort, and overall quality of life.

Airborne Contact Dermatitis

Airborne contact dermatitis is a specialized form of the condition that is triggered by exposure to airborne irritants or allergens, rather than direct skin contact. This type of contact dermatitis can be particularly challenging to identify and manage, as the offending triggers may not be immediately apparent.

Causes and Triggers

Airborne contact dermatitis can be triggered by a variety of airborne substances, including:

- Plant-based allergens: Pollen, spores, and other plant-derived particles can trigger airborne ACD in sensitive individuals.

- Industrial and occupational exposures: Certain industrial processes, such as welding or painting, can release airborne irritants or allergens that may lead to airborne contact dermatitis.

- Household chemicals: Vapors or fumes from household cleaners, paints, or other volatile compounds can be potential triggers.
- Medications: Aerosolized medications, such as certain inhalers or nebulizers, may occasionally cause airborne contact dermatitis.

Clinical Presentation

The symptoms of airborne contact dermatitis can vary depending on the specific trigger and the route of exposure, but may include:

- Localized skin lesions: The skin reaction may be confined to the areas of the body that are directly exposed to the airborne trigger, such as the face, neck, or upper extremities.
- Widespread distribution: In some cases, the skin reaction can spread to other areas of the body, even if they were not directly exposed to the trigger.
- Respiratory symptoms: Individuals with airborne contact dermatitis may also experience respiratory symptoms, such as nasal congestion, sneezing, or coughing, due to the inhalation of the offending substance.
- Ocular involvement: The eyes may also be affected, leading to redness, itching, or swelling of the eyelids or conjunctiva.

Diagnosis and Assessment

Diagnosing airborne contact dermatitis can be challenging, as the offending trigger may not be immediately apparent. Healthcare providers will typically begin with a thorough medical history, focusing on the patient's environmental and occupational exposures, as well as any seasonal or temporal patterns to the skin reactions.

Additional diagnostic tests that may be employed include:

- Patch testing: To identify any specific allergens that may be triggering the airborne contact dermatitis.
- Provocation testing: Controlled exposure to suspected triggers, either through inhalation or direct application to the skin, can help confirm the

diagnosis.

  - Environmental assessments: Evaluating the patient's home, workplace, or other relevant environments for the presence of potential airborne irritants or allergens.

Assessing the severity and impact of airborne contact dermatitis is crucial, as this can guide the development of an appropriate management plan. Healthcare providers may use tools such as the Airborne Contact Dermat

CHAPTER 7

Chapter 7: Contact Dermatitis in Children

While contact dermatitis is a common skin condition that can affect individuals of all ages, the presentation and management of this condition in children can pose unique challenges and considerations. Children's developing skin, immune systems, and behavioral patterns can all contribute to the distinct features and management approaches required for pediatric contact dermatitis.

In this chapter, we will explore the specific characteristics, triggers, and diagnostic considerations for contact dermatitis in children. We will also delve into the specialized treatment strategies and preventive measures that healthcare providers and caregivers can employ to effectively manage this skin condition in the pediatric population.

By the end of this chapter, you will have a comprehensive understanding of the unique aspects of contact dermatitis in children, equipping you with the knowledge and tools to work collaboratively with your healthcare team to ensure the best possible outcomes for young patients.

Understanding Pediatric Contact Dermatitis

Contact dermatitis in children can manifest in a similar manner to the condition in adults, with both irritant and allergic subtypes presenting with characteristic skin inflammation, redness, and itching. However, there are several key differences that healthcare providers and caregivers should be aware of when managing this skin condition in the pediatric population.

Unique Triggers and Exposures

Children's environments and behaviors can expose them to a distinct set of potential irritants and allergens that may trigger contact dermatitis:

1. Toys and Playthings:
    - Metals (e.g., nickel in jewelry or metal fasteners)
    - Dyes or chemicals in fabrics, plastics, or paints
    - Latex in balloons or other rubber products

2. Clothing and Fabrics:
    - Dyes, finishes, or chemicals used in textile manufacturing
    - Wool or other coarse, irritating materials
    - Elastic or synthetic fabrics that may cause friction

3. Personal Care Products:
    - Fragrances, preservatives, or other ingredients in baby wipes, soaps, or lotions
    - Ingredients in diaper rash creams or other topical medications

4. Food and Dietary Exposures:
    - Certain foods or food additives that may trigger allergic reactions
    - Contact with raw or uncooked foods during meal preparation

5. Environmental Factors:
    - Outdoor allergens, such as pollen or mold spores
    - Chemicals or irritants in the home, school, or daycare environments

Understanding these unique triggers and exposure patterns is crucial for healthcare providers and caregivers to effectively prevent and manage contact dermatitis in children.

Developmental Considerations
The developing nature of a child's skin and immune system can also impact the presentation and management of contact dermatitis:

1. Skin Barrier Function:
   - Children, especially infants, have a less developed stratum corneum, making their skin more vulnerable to irritants and allergens.
   - Frequent bathing, diaper use, and other environmental exposures can further compromise the skin's barrier function in young children.

2. Immune System Maturation:
   - A child's immune system continues to develop and mature, which can affect their susceptibility to allergic contact dermatitis.
   - Certain allergens may trigger more severe reactions in children compared to adults.

3. Behavioral Factors:
   - Children's natural curiosity and tendency to explore their environment can increase their exposure to potential irritants and allergens.
   - Increased hand-to-mouth and hand-to-eye behaviors in young children can facilitate the transfer of triggers to sensitive areas.

Recognizing these developmental factors is crucial for healthcare providers and caregivers to implement appropriate prevention strategies and tailor the management of contact dermatitis in children.

Diagnosing Contact Dermatitis in Children

The diagnostic process for contact dermatitis in children often follows a similar approach to that used in adults, but with some specialized considerations:

Medical History and Physical Examination

When evaluating a child with suspected contact dermatitis, healthcare providers will gather a detailed medical history, focusing on the following key elements:

- Onset and duration of the skin condition
    - Potential triggers or exposures, including toys, clothing, personal care products, and environmental factors
    - Family history of atopic dermatitis or other allergic conditions
    - Previous treatments and response to interventions

The physical examination will involve a careful assessment of the child's skin, looking for characteristic signs of contact dermatitis, such as redness, swelling, vesicles, and eczematous changes. Healthcare providers may also evaluate the distribution and pattern of the skin lesions to help differentiate between irritant and allergic subtypes.

Diagnostic Testing

In some cases, healthcare providers may recommend additional diagnostic tests to confirm the diagnosis and identify the specific trigger or allergen responsible for the child's contact dermatitis:

1. Patch testing: This specialized procedure involves the controlled application of a series of known allergens to the child's skin, typically on the back. Patch testing can help identify the specific allergens that are triggering the skin reaction, though it may require adaptation for the pediatric population.

2. Skin biopsy: A small sample of the affected skin may be collected and analyzed under a microscope to help distinguish contact dermatitis from other skin conditions and provide insight into the underlying pathology.

3. Allergy testing: For children with suspected allergic contact dermatitis, additional allergy testing, such as blood tests or intradermal skin tests, may

be performed to identify the specific allergens involved.

It is important to note that the interpretation and performance of these diagnostic tests in children may require specialized expertise and tailored protocols to ensure the safety and comfort of the young patient.

Managing Contact Dermatitis in Children

The management of contact dermatitis in children often involves a combination of topical treatments, systemic therapies, and preventive strategies, with a focus on addressing the unique needs and considerations of the pediatric population.

Topical Treatments

Topical therapies continue to play a central role in the management of contact dermatitis in children, but healthcare providers must carefully consider the appropriate potency and formulations to ensure safety and efficacy:

1. Topical corticosteroids:
   - Healthcare providers may prescribe low- to medium-potency topical corticosteroids to help reduce inflammation and alleviate symptoms.
   - The use of topical corticosteroids in children requires close monitoring to minimize the risk of adverse effects, such as skin thinning or growth suppression.

2. Topical calcineurin inhibitors:
   - These immunomodulatory agents may be used in the management of chronic or recalcitrant pediatric contact dermatitis, as they can help modulate the underlying immune response without the risk of skin thinning.
   - Careful dosing and monitoring are necessary to ensure the safety and effectiveness of these medications in children.

3. Emollients and barrier creams:
   - Gentle, fragrance-free moisturizers and barrier creams can help restore the skin's protective function and prevent further irritation or allergen exposure.
   - These products are often well-tolerated and can be an important component of the management plan for pediatric contact dermatitis.

Systemic Treatments

In some cases of severe or widespread pediatric contact dermatitis, healthcare providers may recommend the use of systemic (oral or injectable) medications to complement the topical management approach:

1. Oral antihistamines:
   - Oral antihistamines can be a valuable adjunct to topical treatments, particularly in the management of allergic contact dermatitis, as they can help alleviate symptoms like itching and swelling.
   - Healthcare providers must carefully consider the appropriate dosage and formulation for the child's age and weight.

2. Oral corticosteroids:
   - For severe or recalcitrant cases of pediatric contact dermatitis that are not responding to topical treatments, a short course of oral corticosteroids may be prescribed to rapidly reduce inflammation and provide relief.
   - The use of systemic corticosteroids in children requires close monitoring and a well-designed tapering plan to minimize the risk of adverse effects.

3. Immunosuppressant drugs:
   - In rare, treatment-resistant cases of pediatric contact dermatitis, healthcare providers may consider the use of systemic immunosuppressant medications, such as cyclosporine or methotrexate, to suppress the underlying immune response.
   - The use of these medications in children requires specialized expertise and careful monitoring to ensure the best possible outcomes.

Preventive Strategies and Patient/Caregiver Education
In addition to medical treatments, the management of contact dermatitis in children often involves a focus on preventive strategies and comprehensive patient/caregiver education:

1. Identification and avoidance of triggers:
   - Helping the child and their caregivers identify and consistently avoid the specific irritants or allergens responsible for the skin condition is crucial for preventing future flare-ups.
   - This may involve modifications to the child's environment, personal care routines, and/or dietary exposures.

2. Gentle skin care practices:
   - Encouraging the use of fragrance-free, hypoallergenic cleansers, moisturizers, and other personal care products can help strengthen the child's skin barrier and prevent further irritation.
   - Providing guidance on appropriate bathing, diapering, and clothing choices can also contribute to the overall skin health of the child.

3. Patient/caregiver education and empowerment:
   - Comprehensive education about the nature of the child's condition, the importance of trigger avoidance, and the proper use of prescribed treatments can help empower caregivers to become active partners in the management process.
   - Providing resources and support for managing the emotional and psychosocial impacts of the condition can also be beneficial for the child and their family.

By adopting a holistic, patient-centered approach to the management of contact dermatitis in children, healthcare providers can work collaboratively with caregivers to achieve the best possible outcomes and promote the long-term skin health and well-being of young patients.

Considerations for Specific Pediatric Populations

While the general management principles for contact dermatitis in children apply across the board, there are some unique considerations for certain pediatric populations that healthcare providers should be aware of:

Infants and Toddlers
Infants and toddlers have particularly vulnerable and developing skin, which can increase their susceptibility to contact dermatitis. Healthcare providers may need to:

- Carefully select age-appropriate, gentle topical treatments with minimal risk of systemic absorption.
    - Closely monitor for any signs of skin irritation or sensitivity to personal care products or other environmental exposures.
    - Provide guidance on appropriate diapering and skin care practices to support the maturation of the infant's skin barrier.

School-age Children
As children enter school and participate in various activities, their exposure to potential irritants and allergens may increase. Healthcare providers may need to:

- Collaborate with school nurses and educators to ensure appropriate accommodations and trigger avoidance strategies are in place.
    - Provide guidance on packing safe, allergy-friendly lunches and snacks for the school environment.
    - Educate children on the importance of avoiding sharing personal items, such as art supplies or sports equipment, that may be contaminated with triggers.

Adolescents
Adolescents may face unique challenges, such as increased use of personal

care products, exposure to new materials (e.g., jewelry, makeup), and heightened self-consciousness about their skin condition. Healthcare providers may need to:

- Address the emotional and psychosocial impacts of contact dermatitis, including the potential for bullying or social isolation.
    - Provide guidance on safe and appropriate personal care routines, including the selection of low-risk cosmetics and skincare products.
    - Encourage open communication and collaboration with the adolescent patient to ensure the management plan aligns with their needs and preferences.

By recognizing and addressing the specific considerations for these diverse pediatric populations, healthcare providers can tailor their approach to the management of contact dermatitis and ensure the best possible outcomes for young patients and their families.

Conclusion

In this chapter, we have explored the unique aspects of contact dermatitis in children, highlighting the distinct triggers, developmental considerations, and specialized management strategies required for this patient population.

Understanding the specialized triggers and exposures that can lead to contact dermatitis in children, as well as the unique characteristics of their developing skin and immune systems, is crucial for healthcare providers to effectively prevent, diagnose, and manage this condition in the pediatric setting.

The comprehensive approach to managing contact dermatitis in children involves a combination of topical and systemic treatments, along with a strong emphasis on preventive strategies and patient/caregiver education. By working collaboratively with families and addressing the holistic needs of young patients, healthcare providers can help children with contact dermatitis achieve optimal skin health and quality of life.

As you continue your journey through this comprehensive guide, the next chapter will focus on the unique considerations and management approaches for contact dermatitis in the occupational setting, empowering you with the specialized knowledge needed to navigate this challenging aspect of the condition.

CHAPTER 8

C hapter 8: Occupational Contact Dermatitis

Occupational contact dermatitis is a significant concern for both workers and employers, posing substantial challenges in terms of lost productivity, healthcare costs, and overall worker well-being. As one of the most common work-related skin diseases, occupational contact dermatitis requires specialized knowledge and a multifaceted approach to prevention, diagnosis, and management.

In this chapter, we will delve into the unique characteristics and considerations surrounding occupational contact dermatitis. We will explore the high-risk professions and industries, the common triggers and exposures, and the key diagnostic and management strategies that healthcare providers and employers can employ to address this occupational health issue.

By the end of this chapter, you will have a comprehensive understanding of the complexities of occupational contact dermatitis, equipping you with the knowledge and tools to work collaboratively with healthcare providers, occupational health specialists, and employers to ensure the best possible outcomes for affected workers.

The Impact of Occupational Contact Dermatitis

Occupational contact dermatitis is a significant and widespread issue, accounting for up to 30% of all work-related skin diseases. The impact of this condition can be far-reaching, affecting both the individual worker and the employer.

Individual Impact

For the worker, occupational contact dermatitis can have a profound impact on their physical, emotional, and financial well-being:

1. Physical Symptoms:
   - Persistent skin inflammation, redness, and itching can lead to significant discomfort and impairment in daily activities.
   - In severe cases, the skin may develop blisters, fissures, or eczematous lesions, further exacerbating the physical symptoms.

2. Functional Limitations:
   - The skin condition can interfere with the worker's ability to perform their job duties, particularly in professions that involve frequent hand use or contact with potential triggers.
   - Prolonged exposure to irritants or allergens can lead to the development of chronic, recurrent forms of contact dermatitis, further compromising the worker's functionality.

3. Emotional and Psychosocial Impacts:
   - The visible nature of contact dermatitis can lead to feelings of embarrassment, self-consciousness, and social isolation, negatively impacting the worker's mental health and overall quality of life.
   - The burden of managing the condition, including the need for frequent medical appointments and treatment regimens, can also contribute to increased stress and anxiety.

4. Financial Consequences:
   - Occupational contact dermatitis can result in lost work days, reduced productivity, and the potential need for job changes or even disability, leading

to significant financial strain for the affected worker.

- In addition, the costs associated with medical treatment and ongoing management of the condition can further exacerbate the financial burden.

Employer and Societal Impact

Occupational contact dermatitis also has significant implications for employers and society as a whole:

1. Productivity and Absenteeism:

- Workers with occupational contact dermatitis may experience increased absenteeism, reduced productivity, and the need for job modifications or changes, all of which can have a substantial impact on the employer's operations and bottom line.

2. Healthcare Costs:

- The management of occupational contact dermatitis, including diagnostic testing, ongoing treatment, and rehabilitation, can lead to significant healthcare expenditures for employers, workers' compensation systems, and the broader healthcare system.

3. Regulatory and Legal Implications:

- In many countries, occupational contact dermatitis is recognized as an occupational disease, which can have implications for workers' compensation, workplace safety regulations, and employer-employee relationships.

4. Societal Burden:

- The cumulative impact of occupational contact dermatitis on individual workers, employers, and the healthcare system can contribute to a significant societal burden, both in terms of economic costs and the overall well-being of the workforce.

Understanding the far-reaching consequences of occupational contact dermatitis is crucial for healthcare providers, employers, and policymakers to develop and implement effective prevention and management strategies that address this critical occupational health issue.

High-Risk Professions and Exposures

Certain occupations and industries are associated with a higher risk of developing occupational contact dermatitis due to the nature of their work and the potential exposures to irritants and allergens.

High-Risk Professions
Some of the professions and industries with the highest rates of occupational contact dermatitis include:

1. Healthcare Workers:
   - Nurses, physicians, laboratory technicians, and other healthcare professionals are at risk of developing contact dermatitis due to frequent exposure to latex, disinfectants, soaps, and other chemicals.

2. Industrial Workers:
   - Individuals working in manufacturing, construction, metalworking, and other industrial settings are often exposed to a wide range of irritants and allergens, including solvents, oils, metals, and mineral dusts.

3. Service Workers:
   - Professions such as hairstylists, beauticians, and food service workers can be prone to contact dermatitis due to their exposure to various chemicals, personal care products, and food-related allergens.

4. Mechanics and Technicians:
   - Workers in the automotive, machinery, and electronics industries may encounter contact dermatitis from exposure to oils, greases, solvents, and metals.

5. Cleaning and Maintenance Workers:
   - Individuals responsible for cleaning and maintaining facilities, such as custodians and janitors, can develop contact dermatitis from exposure to disinfectants, detergents, and other cleaning agents.

Common Exposures and Triggers
The specific triggers and exposures that can lead to occupational contact dermatitis vary depending on the profession and work environment, but often include:

1. Chemicals and Solvents:
   - Acids, alkalis, degreasers, and other corrosive or irritating chemicals commonly used in industrial and manufacturing settings.

2. Metals:
   - Nickel, chromium, cobalt, and other metallic compounds found in tools, machinery, and various industrial processes.

3. Rubber and Latex:
   - Natural rubber latex, used in gloves and other medical devices, can trigger allergic reactions in sensitized individuals, particularly healthcare workers.

4. Personal Care Products:
   - Fragrances, preservatives, and other ingredients in hair products, cosmetics, and skin care items used by service workers.

5. Food and Food-Related Allergens:
   - Proteins, enzymes, and other food-related substances that can trigger allergic reactions in food service and processing workers.

6. Wet Work and Occlusion:
   - Prolonged exposure to water, moisture, and occlusive clothing or equipment, which can compromise the skin's barrier function and lead to

irritant contact dermatitis.

Recognizing these high-risk professions and common exposures is crucial for healthcare providers, employers, and occupational health specialists to develop targeted prevention strategies and early intervention measures to address occupational contact dermatitis.

Unique Challenges in Occupational Settings

Occupational contact dermatitis poses several unique challenges compared to non-occupational cases, requiring a specialized and multifaceted approach to management.

Continuous Exposure

One of the primary challenges in occupational settings is the continuous or repeated exposure to potential irritants and allergens. Unlike individuals who may only encounter a trigger in their personal or home environment, workers in high-risk professions often face daily or even hourly exposures to the substances that can lead to the development of contact dermatitis.

This continuous exposure can make it significantly more challenging to identify and eliminate the specific trigger, as the worker may not have the option to simply avoid the offending substance. It also increases the risk of the condition becoming chronic or recurrent, as the skin is repeatedly subjected to the damaging effects of the irritant or allergen.

Financial Implications

The financial impact of occupational contact dermatitis can be substantial, both for the individual worker and the employer. Lost work days, reduced productivity, and the potential need for job changes or even permanent disability can lead to significant economic burdens, including:

- Reduced income and earning potential for the affected worker

- Increased healthcare costs for the management of the condition
- Workers' compensation claims and associated expenses for the employer
- Indirect costs, such as the need for training and replacement of affected workers

These financial implications can create substantial challenges for both the worker and the employer, potentially leading to conflicts, reduced worker morale, and even legal disputes.

Regulatory Considerations

In many countries, occupational contact dermatitis is recognized as an occupational disease, which can have important implications for workers' compensation, workplace safety regulations, and employer-employee relationships. Healthcare providers, employers, and workers must navigate the complex web of regulatory requirements and reporting obligations to ensure compliance and access to appropriate benefits and support.

These regulatory considerations can add an additional layer of complexity to the management of occupational contact dermatitis, requiring close collaboration between healthcare providers, occupational health specialists, and regulatory authorities.

Diagnostic Challenges

Accurately diagnosing the specific cause of occupational contact dermatitis can be more complex compared to non-occupational cases. Workers in high-risk professions may be exposed to multiple potential triggers in their work environment, making it challenging to pinpoint the exact substance or combination of substances responsible for the skin reaction.

Additionally, the continuous exposure and repeated episodes of contact dermatitis can lead to more atypical or overlapping symptoms, further complicating the diagnostic process. Healthcare providers must be equipped with specialized knowledge and diagnostic tools, such as detailed occupational histories and targeted patch testing, to effectively identify the underlying cause of the condition.

Addressing these unique challenges in occupational settings requires a multidisciplinary approach, involving close collaboration between health-care providers, employers, occupational health specialists, and regulatory authorities to ensure the best possible outcomes for affected workers.

Diagnostic and Management Strategies

Effectively addressing occupational contact dermatitis requires a comprehensive, evidence-based approach that combines accurate diagnosis, targeted treatment, and proactive prevention strategies.

Comprehensive Evaluation
The diagnostic process for occupational contact dermatitis often begins with a thorough evaluation, including:

1. Detailed Occupational History:
   - Gathering information about the worker's job duties, work environment, and potential exposures to irritants and allergens.
   - Assessing the temporal relationship between the worker's exposures and the development or exacerbation of skin symptoms.

2. Physical Examination:
   - Carefully examining the affected skin and evaluating the pattern, distribution, and characteristics of the skin lesions.
   - Considering the potential for overlapping or atypical presentations due to the continuous nature of the exposure.

3. Diagnostic Testing:
   - Performing patch testing to identify the specific allergens responsible for the worker's skin reaction.

- Considering additional tests, such as skin biopsies or specialized allergy assessments, in cases where the diagnosis is unclear.

By conducting a comprehensive evaluation, healthcare providers can accurately identify the underlying cause of the occupational contact dermatitis and develop an appropriate management plan.

Targeted Treatment Approaches

The management of occupational contact dermatitis typically involves a combination of topical and systemic therapies, as well as workplace-specific interventions:

1. Topical Treatments:
   - Prescribing appropriate topical corticosteroids, calcineurin inhibitors, or barrier creams to address the skin's inflammatory response.
   - Ensuring the selected products are well-tolerated and do not further exacerbate the worker's skin condition.

2. Systemic Therapies:
   - Utilizing oral antihistamines, corticosteroids, or immunosuppressant medications in severe or recalcitrant cases, under close medical supervision.
   - Carefully managing the potential side effects and monitoring the worker's response to these systemic treatments.

3. Workplace Interventions:
   - Recommending engineering controls, such as ventilation or containment systems, to minimize the worker's exposure to irritants and allergens.
   - Suggesting the use of personal protective equipment (PPE), such as gloves or protective clothing, to create a barrier between the worker's skin and the trigger.
   - Providing guidance on appropriate work practices and hygiene routines to support the management of the condition.

By employing a tailored, multifaceted approach to treatment, healthcare providers can help the affected worker manage their symptoms, prevent the progression of the condition, and maintain their ability to perform their job duties.

Comprehensive Prevention Strategies

Effective prevention of occupational contact dermatitis requires a collaborative effort between healthcare providers, employers, and occupational health specialists. Key prevention strategies may include:

1. Workplace Assessments:
   - Conducting comprehensive evaluations of the work environment to identify potential sources of irritants and allergens.
   - Implementing engineering controls, substituting hazardous materials, and improving work practices to minimize exposure risks.

2. Worker Education and Training:
   - Providing comprehensive education to workers on the recognition, prevention, and management of occupational contact dermatitis.
   - Empowering workers to identify and report potential triggers, as well as to adopt appropriate skin care and protective measures.

3. Screening and Early Intervention:
   - Implementing regular skin screenings and health monitoring programs to facilitate the early detection and management of occupational contact dermatitis.
   - Ensuring prompt and effective treatment to prevent the condition from becoming chronic or recurrent.

4. Collaborative Approach:
   - Fostering a collaborative partnership between healthcare providers, employers, and occupational health specialists to develop and implement comprehensive prevention strategies.

- Ensuring clear communication, shared decision-making, and ongoing monitoring to optimize the effectiveness of the prevention program.

By adopting a proactive, multifaceted approach to prevention, healthcare providers, employers, and occupational health specialists can work together to mitigate the impact of occupational contact dermatitis and promote the long-term health and well-being of the workforce.

Navigating Workers' Compensation

In many countries, occupational contact dermatitis is recognized as an occupational disease, which can have important implications for workers' compensation and the management of the condition.

Establishing the Causal Relationship
One of the key challenges in the workers' compensation process is establishing a clear causal relationship between the worker's occupational exposures and the development of contact dermatitis. Healthcare providers play a crucial role in this process, as they must document the worker's medical history, occupational exposures, and the timeline of symptom development to support the claim.

Detailed medical records, job-site evaluations, and, in some cases, specialized diagnostic testing can all contribute to the evidence needed to substantiate the causal link between the worker's condition and their occupation.

Navigating the Workers' Compensation System
Once the causal relationship has been established, the worker must navigate the complex workers' compensation system to access the necessary benefits and support. This may involve:

1. Filing the Appropriate Claims:
   - Submitting the necessary documentation and paperwork to the relevant

workers' compensation authorities.
   - Ensuring compliance with all reporting requirements and deadlines.

2. Accessing Approved Healthcare Providers:
   - Identifying and utilizing healthcare providers who are authorized to treat workers' compensation cases.
   - Coordinating the management of the occupational contact dermatitis with the approved providers.

3. Securing Appropriate Benefits:
   - Obtaining coverage for medical treatment, including diagnostic testing, therapies, and any necessary work accommodations or modifications.
   - Accessing wage replacement or disability benefits, if the worker is unable to perform their job duties due to the occupational condition.

4. Maintaining Clear Communication:
   - Fostering open dialogue with the workers' compensation authorities, employers, and healthcare providers to ensure a smooth and effective process.
   - Addressing any challenges or disputes that may arise during the claims process.

By understanding the workers' compensation system and working collaboratively with healthcare providers and occupational health specialists, affected workers can navigate the complexities of occupational contact dermatitis and access the necessary support and benefits to facilitate their recovery and return to work.

Conclusion

In this chapter, we have explored the unique challenges and considerations surrounding occupational contact dermatitis, a significant and often overlooked occupational health issue.

We have discussed the profound impact that occupational contact dermatitis can have on individual workers, employers, and society as a whole, highlighting the need for a comprehensive, multifaceted approach to prevention, diagnosis, and management.

By recognizing the high-risk professions and common exposures associated with occupational contact dermatitis, healthcare providers, employers, and occupational health specialists can work collaboratively to develop targeted strategies that address the unique challenges of this condition in the workplace setting.

Importantly, we have also emphasized the crucial role of accurate diagnosis, tailored treatment approaches, and proactive prevention measures in minimizing the burden of occupational contact dermatitis. Additionally, we have explored the complexities of navigating the workers' compensation system, underscoring the importance of clear communication, documentation, and collaborative efforts to ensure the best possible outcomes for affected workers.

As you continue your journey through this comprehensive guide, the next chapter will delve into the specialized diagnostic tools and techniques used to identify the specific triggers and allergens responsible for contact dermatitis, empowering you with the knowledge to partner with healthcare providers and guide the diagnostic process.

CHAPTER 9

Chapter 9: Patch Testing and Allergen Identification

Accurately identifying the specific triggers and allergens responsible for a patient's contact dermatitis is a critical step in developing an effective management plan. While the clinical presentation and medical history can provide valuable insights, the use of specialized diagnostic tools, such as patch testing, is often necessary to pinpoint the underlying cause of the skin condition.

In this chapter, we will explore the purpose and methodology of patch testing, the interpretation of results, and the importance of avoiding future exposures to the identified allergens. By understanding the role of patch testing and other diagnostic approaches, patients and healthcare providers can work collaboratively to uncover the root causes of contact dermatitis and implement targeted strategies to achieve the best possible outcomes.

The Purpose of Patch Testing

Patch testing is a widely recognized diagnostic tool used to identify the specific allergens that are triggering a patient's allergic contact dermatitis (ACD). This procedure involves the controlled application of a series of known allergens to the patient's skin, allowing healthcare providers to determine which substances the individual has developed a sensitivity to.

The primary goals of patch testing in the context of contact dermatitis are:

1. Allergen Identification:
   - Patch testing helps healthcare providers identify the specific allergens responsible for the patient's skin condition, whether it is a single trigger or a combination of multiple allergens.
   - This information is crucial for developing targeted avoidance strategies and guiding the overall management of the patient's ACD.

2. Confirmation of Diagnosis:
   - Positive patch test results can provide objective evidence to support the diagnosis of ACD, particularly in cases where the clinical presentation alone is not sufficient to differentiate it from other skin conditions.

3. Ruling Out Potential Triggers:
   - Patch testing can also help rule out certain allergens as the cause of the patient's skin condition, allowing healthcare providers to focus their efforts on identifying the true trigger(s).

4. Guiding Treatment Decisions:
   - The results of patch testing can inform the selection of appropriate topical and systemic treatments, as well as the implementation of effective prevention strategies.

By employing patch testing as part of the diagnostic process, healthcare providers can obtain the necessary information to tailor the management of ACD to the individual patient's specific needs and allergic profile.

Patch Testing Methodology

Patch testing is typically performed by healthcare providers with specialized training and expertise in this diagnostic procedure, such as dermatologists or allergists. The process generally involves the following steps:

1. Allergen Selection:

- Healthcare providers will select a standard series of known contact allergens to apply to the patient's skin, based on the patient's medical history, occupational exposures, and the most common triggers for ACD.

- The specific allergens tested may include metals (e.g., nickel, cobalt, chromium), fragrances, preservatives, rubber chemicals, and plant-based substances (e.g., urushiol from poison ivy).

- In some cases, healthcare providers may also test additional, patient-specific allergens based on the individual's suspected triggers.

2. Patch Application:

- Small amounts of the selected allergens are applied to the patient's back, typically using standardized patch test chambers or strips.

- The patches are left in place for a specific duration, usually between 48 and 72 hours, to allow for the development of any skin reactions.

3. Observation and Scoring:

- During the patch test application and at subsequent follow-up appointments, the healthcare provider will carefully examine the skin for any signs of a reaction, such as redness, swelling, or the formation of vesicles.

- The severity of the reaction is typically scored using a standardized grading scale, with higher scores indicating a stronger allergic response.

4. Interpretation of Results:

- Based on the scoring of the patch test reactions, the healthcare provider will determine which allergens the patient has tested positive for, indicating a true allergic sensitivity.

- The interpretation of patch test results requires specialized knowledge and experience to ensure accurate identification of the relevant allergens.

It is important to note that patch testing is generally considered a safe and well-tolerated diagnostic procedure, with a low risk of adverse reactions. However, healthcare providers must still take appropriate precautions and ensure the patient's comfort throughout the process.

Interpreting Patch Test Results

The interpretation of patch test results is a critical step in the diagnostic process, as it enables healthcare providers to identify the specific allergens responsible for the patient's ACD and guide the development of a targeted management plan.

Positive Patch Test Reactions

A positive patch test reaction is typically characterized by the development of redness, swelling, and/or the formation of vesicles or eczematous changes at the site where the allergen was applied. The severity of the reaction is often graded using a standardized scale, such as the International Contact Dermatitis Research Group (ICDRG) scoring system:

- + (weak positive reaction): Erythema, infiltration, possibly papules
  - ++ (strong positive reaction): Erythema, infiltration, papules, vesicles
  - +++ (extreme positive reaction): Intense erythema, infiltration, coalescing vesicles

A positive patch test reaction indicates that the patient has developed a true allergic sensitivity to the tested allergen and is likely to experience a similar skin reaction upon future exposure.

Negative Patch Test Reactions

If a patient does not exhibit any visible reaction to a specific allergen during the patch test, the result is considered negative. A negative patch test result suggests that the patient does not have an allergic sensitivity to that particular substance.

It is important to note that a negative patch test does not necessarily rule out the possibility of the allergen being responsible for the patient's ACD. Some factors, such as the specific formulation of the allergen, the timing of the test, or the patient's individual sensitivity, can influence the test results.

Relevance of Patch Test Findings

Even when a positive patch test result is obtained, it is crucial for healthcare providers to determine the clinical relevance of the allergen in the patient's specific case. Factors to consider include:

- Temporal relationship: Is there a clear association between the patient's exposure to the allergen and the development or exacerbation of their skin condition?
    - Exposure patterns: How often and in what contexts is the patient likely to encounter the identified allergen?
    - Avoidance strategies: Is it feasible for the patient to consistently avoid the allergen in their daily life and work environment?

By carefully evaluating the relevance of the patch test findings, healthcare providers can work with the patient to develop an effective management plan that addresses the specific allergens contributing to their ACD.

Avoiding Future Exposures

Once the specific allergens responsible for a patient's ACD have been identified through patch testing, the next critical step is to implement strategies to avoid future exposure to these triggers. This is essential for preventing the recurrence or exacerbation of the skin condition and promoting long-term management success.

Identifying Potential Sources of Exposure

To effectively avoid the identified allergens, patients and healthcare providers must first work together to determine all potential sources of exposure. This may involve:

- Reviewing the patient's medical and exposure history in detail
   - Conducting a thorough assessment of the patient's home, work, and recreational environments
   - Carefully examining the ingredients in personal care products, household items, and consumer goods
   - Identifying any occupational or hobby-related activities that may involve exposure to the allergen

By mapping out the various ways the patient may encounter the allergen, healthcare providers can develop a comprehensive avoidance plan tailored to the individual's specific needs and lifestyle.

Implementing Avoidance Strategies
   Once the potential sources of exposure have been identified, patients can begin implementing strategies to minimize or eliminate contact with the identified allergens. These strategies may include:

1. Product Substitution:
   - Replacing personal care products, household items, and other consumer goods that contain the identified allergens with alternative, hypoallergenic options.
   - Carefully reading ingredient labels to avoid products that may trigger a reaction.

2. Workplace Modifications:
   - Collaborating with employers to implement engineering controls, such as ventilation or containment systems, to reduce exposure in the workplace.
   - Utilizing personal protective equipment (PPE), such as gloves or protective clothing, to create a barrier between the skin and the allergen.
   - Exploring the possibility of job modifications or reassignment to minimize exposure, if necessary.

3. Lifestyle Adjustments:

- Avoiding activities or hobbies that may involve exposure to the identified allergens.

- Replacing or modifying materials used in recreational pursuits (e.g., substituting non-latex gloves for certain sports or crafts).

- Implementing protective measures during travel or other activities where exposure may occur.

4. Comprehensive Patient Education:
- Providing patients with detailed information about the identified allergens, including their common uses and sources of exposure.

- Empowering patients to become active partners in the avoidance process, equipping them with the knowledge and skills to identify and eliminate triggers.

- Encouraging patients to maintain detailed exposure logs and report any potential exposures or symptom exacerbations to their healthcare providers.

By working closely with their healthcare team to implement a comprehensive avoidance plan, patients can significantly reduce their risk of future allergic reactions and promote the long-term management of their ACD.

Ongoing Monitoring and Follow-up

Effectively avoiding the identified allergens is a crucial component of the management strategy for ACD, but it is not a one-time event. Ongoing monitoring and follow-up care are essential to ensure the continued effectiveness of the avoidance plan and to address any new challenges that may arise.

Regular check-ins with the healthcare provider, whether in person or through virtual visits, can help track the patient's progress, assess the efficacy of the avoidance strategies, and make any necessary adjustments to the management plan. During these follow-up appointments, the healthcare provider may:

1. Evaluate the patient's skin condition and monitor for any changes or new developments.
2. Discuss any new exposures or potential triggers that the patient has encountered and provide advice on how to avoid or mitigate them.
3. Order additional diagnostic tests, such as repeat patch testing or allergy evaluations, if warranted by the patient's evolving condition or new exposures.
4. Collaborate with the patient to refine the avoidance plan, address any challenges or concerns, and set realistic goals for maintaining long-term skin health.

Fostering a collaborative partnership between the patient and the healthcare provider is crucial for the successful long-term management of ACD. By working together, they can navigate the complexities of allergen avoidance, optimize treatment outcomes, and empower the patient to take an active role in managing their skin health.

Conclusion

In this chapter, we have explored the critical role of patch testing and allergen identification in the management of contact dermatitis, particularly the allergic subtype. By understanding the purpose and methodology of this specialized diagnostic procedure, as well as the interpretation of the results, patients and healthcare providers can work collaboratively to uncover the specific triggers responsible for the skin condition.

Identifying the relevant allergens is just the first step, as the next crucial task is to implement effective strategies to avoid future exposures. We have discussed the importance of mapping out potential sources of exposure, developing comprehensive avoidance plans, and empowering patients with the knowledge and skills to become active partners in their own care.

Ongoing monitoring and follow-up care are essential to ensure the continued effectiveness of the avoidance strategies and to address any new challenges that may arise over time. By fostering a collaborative relationship between the patient and the healthcare provider, individuals with ACD can achieve the best possible outcomes and maintain long-term control over their skin health.

As you continue your journey through this comprehensive guide, the next chapter will focus on the various topical and systemic treatment options available for the management of contact dermatitis, equipping you with the knowledge to develop personalized, evidence-based treatment plans that address the unique needs of each patient.

CHAPTER 10

Chapter 10: Topical Treatments for Contact Dermatitis

Topical therapies play a central role in the management of contact dermatitis, whether the condition is triggered by irritants or allergens. These localized treatments are often the first line of defense in addressing the skin's inflammatory response and promoting healing, and they can be an essential component of a comprehensive treatment plan.

In this chapter, we will explore the various topical treatment options available for the management of contact dermatitis, including corticosteroids, calcineurin inhibitors, and barrier creams/emollients. We will delve into the mechanisms of action, appropriate usage, and potential side effects of these topical treatments, empowering both patients and healthcare providers to make informed decisions and achieve the best possible outcomes.

By understanding the strengths and limitations of each topical therapy, you will be better equipped to work collaboratively with your healthcare team to develop personalized treatment strategies that address the specific needs and characteristics of your contact dermatitis.

Topical Corticosteroids

Topical corticosteroids are the mainstay of treatment for both irritant and allergic contact dermatitis, and they are widely considered the most effective topical option for addressing the skin's inflammatory response.

Mechanism of Action
Topical corticosteroids work by reducing the production and activity of various inflammatory mediators, such as cytokines, prostaglandins, and leukotrienes, which play a central role in the development and perpetuation of the skin's inflammatory reaction. By targeting these key components of the inflammatory cascade, topical corticosteroids can help alleviate the characteristic symptoms of contact dermatitis, including redness, swelling, and itching.

Topical Corticosteroid Potencies
Topical corticosteroids are available in a range of potencies, from low-strength (e.g., hydrocortisone) to high-potency (e.g., clobetasol propionate) formulations. The choice of corticosteroid product is based on several factors, including:

- Severity of the skin condition: More severe or extensive cases of contact dermatitis may require higher-potency corticosteroids to effectively control the inflammation.
  - Location of the affected area: Certain body regions, such as the face, intertriginous areas, and thin skin, may be more sensitive and require lower-potency corticosteroids to minimize the risk of adverse effects.
  - Patient age and overall health status: Healthcare providers may select lower-potency corticosteroids for use in pediatric patients or individuals with certain underlying medical conditions.

It is important to note that the prolonged or inappropriate use of high-potency topical corticosteroids can lead to adverse effects, such as skin thinning, striae (stretch marks), and the development of steroid-induced dermatitis. Healthcare providers must carefully weigh the risks and benefits when prescribing these medications and provide clear guidance to patients on their proper use.

Topical Corticosteroid Formulations

Topical corticosteroids are available in a variety of formulations, including creams, ointments, lotions, and gels. The choice of formulation is often based on the specific characteristics of the affected skin and the patient's preferences:

- Creams are generally well-tolerated and readily absorbed, making them a good option for use on most body areas.
  - Ointments are more occlusive and emollient, which can be beneficial for dry, scaly, or lichenified skin.
  - Lotions and gels may be preferred for use on hairy or intertriginous areas, as they are less greasy and more cosmetically elegant.

Patients should be instructed on the appropriate application techniques, such as using the smallest effective amount, avoiding the eyes and mucous membranes, and following the prescribed dosing schedule.

Calcineurin Inhibitors

In addition to topical corticosteroids, another class of topical medications used in the management of contact dermatitis is calcineurin inhibitors, also known as topical immunomodulators.

Mechanism of Action

Calcineurin inhibitors, such as tacrolimus and pimecrolimus, work by disrupting the signaling pathways that drive the allergic inflammatory response. These medications target specific immune cells, known as T cells, which play a central role in the development of allergic contact dermatitis (ACD). By modulating the activity of these T cells, calcineurin inhibitors can help reduce the intensity of the skin's allergic reaction without the risk of skin thinning associated with prolonged corticosteroid use.

Indications for Use

Topical calcineurin inhibitors are primarily indicated for the management of chronic or recalcitrant cases of contact dermatitis, particularly in situations where the use of topical corticosteroids may be problematic or contraindicated, such as:

- Sensitive skin areas (e.g., face, intertriginous regions)
    - Prolonged or continuous treatment requirements
    - Concerns about the potential for skin thinning or other adverse effects with corticosteroids

Healthcare providers may also consider using topical calcineurin inhibitors as a steroid-sparing agent, allowing for the reduction of corticosteroid use while maintaining effective control of the skin's inflammatory response.

Safety Considerations
While topical calcineurin inhibitors are generally well-tolerated, they do carry some potential risks and side effects that healthcare providers and patients should be aware of:

- Transient burning or stinging sensation upon initial application
    - Increased susceptibility to skin infections, particularly during the first few weeks of use
    - Potential for systemic absorption and associated risks, especially with prolonged, widespread, or occlusive use

Healthcare providers must carefully weigh the risks and benefits of using topical calcineurin inhibitors, particularly in certain patient populations, such as children or individuals with compromised immune systems.

Barrier Creams and Emollients

In addition to the anti-inflammatory properties of topical corticosteroids and calcineurin inhibitors, barrier creams and emollient moisturizers also play a crucial role in the management of contact dermatitis.

Restoring Skin Barrier Function
One of the primary mechanisms by which barrier creams and emollients can benefit individuals with contact dermatitis is by helping to restore the skin's protective function. In both irritant and allergic contact dermatitis, the skin's outer layer, known as the stratum corneum, can become compromised, leading to increased permeability and susceptibility to further irritation or allergen exposure.

Barrier creams and emollients work by replenishing the skin's natural lipids and hydrating the stratum corneum, which can help strengthen the skin's barrier and reduce the risk of additional triggers penetrating the skin.

Soothing and Hydrating the Skin
In addition to their barrier-restoring properties, barrier creams and emollients can also provide immediate relief and comfort to the inflamed, itchy skin associated with contact dermatitis. The occlusive and hydrating nature of these products can help soothe the skin, alleviate dryness and scaling, and promote the healing process.

Preventing Further Irritation
By creating a protective layer on the skin's surface, barrier creams and emollients can also help minimize the risk of additional exposure to irritants or allergens. This is particularly important in the management of contact dermatitis, where avoiding the triggering substance is a critical component of the overall treatment strategy.

Selecting Appropriate Formulations
When recommending barrier creams and emollients for patients with contact dermatitis, healthcare providers must consider several factors to ensure the products are well-tolerated and effective:

- Fragrance-free and hypoallergenic: To avoid further irritation or allergic reactions, it is essential to select products that are free of fragrances, preservatives, and other potential irritants.
   - Occlusive and moisturizing: Formulations that are rich in emollient ingredients, such as petrolatum, ceramides, and glycerin, can provide the necessary hydration and barrier protection.
   - Cosmetic elegance: Patients may be more likely to adhere to a treatment regimen if the barrier creams and emollients are easy to apply and do not leave a greasy or heavy residue on the skin.

By incorporating barrier creams and emollients into the management plan for contact dermatitis, healthcare providers can provide comprehensive, synergistic care that addresses the skin's inflammatory response, promotes healing, and prevents further exacerbations.

Topical Treatment Considerations

When prescribing and using topical treatments for contact dermatitis, both healthcare providers and patients should be aware of several important considerations to ensure the best possible outcomes.

Proper Application Techniques
   Ensuring the correct application of topical medications is crucial for their effectiveness and to minimize the risk of adverse effects. Healthcare providers should provide clear instructions to patients on the appropriate:

- Amount of product to use (e.g., "pea-sized" for the face, "fingertip unit" for larger areas)
   - Frequency of application (e.g., once or twice daily)
   - Methods of application (e.g., gentle rubbing, avoiding sensitive areas)
   - Duration of treatment (e.g., based on the severity and response)

Educating patients on proper application techniques can help improve adherence and maximize the benefits of the topical therapies.

Monitoring for Side Effects
While topical treatments for contact dermatitis are generally well-tolerated, there are some potential side effects that healthcare providers and patients should be aware of and monitor for:

- Topical corticosteroids: Potential side effects include skin thinning, striae, telangiectasia (visible blood vessels), and the development of steroid-induced dermatitis.
- Topical calcineurin inhibitors: Potential side effects include a transient burning or stinging sensation, increased susceptibility to infections, and the rare risk of systemic absorption.
- Barrier creams and emollients: Potential side effects are generally minimal, but patients should be monitored for any signs of worsening irritation or allergic reaction.

Patients should be instructed to report any concerning side effects to their healthcare provider, who can then make appropriate adjustments to the treatment plan.

Coordination with Systemic Therapies
In some cases of contact dermatitis, particularly in severe or recalcitrant cases, topical treatments may be used in conjunction with systemic (oral or injectable) medications to provide more comprehensive management. Healthcare providers must carefully coordinate the use of topical and systemic therapies, ensuring that they are compatible, effectively address the underlying condition, and do not result in any adverse interactions or compounding side effects.

Adherence and Persistence
Successful management of contact dermatitis often requires consistent and long-term use of topical treatments. Healthcare providers should emphasize

the importance of adherence to the prescribed regimen, as inconsistent or premature discontinuation of topical therapies can lead to suboptimal outcomes and the potential for recurrence or exacerbation of the skin condition.

By addressing these key considerations and working collaboratively with patients, healthcare providers can optimize the use of topical treatments and ensure the best possible outcomes in the management of contact dermatitis.

Conclusion

In this chapter, we have explored the essential role of topical treatments in the management of contact dermatitis, including the use of corticosteroids, calcineurin inhibitors, and barrier creams/emollients. Understanding the mechanisms of action, appropriate usage, and potential side effects of these topical therapies is crucial for both healthcare providers and patients to develop effective, personalized treatment plans.

Topical corticosteroids remain the mainstay of treatment, providing potent anti-inflammatory effects to address the skin's reaction. Calcineurin inhibitors, on the other hand, offer a steroid-sparing alternative for long-term management, particularly in sensitive areas or for chronic cases. Barrier creams and emollients play a complementary role, helping to restore the skin's protective function and prevent further irritation or allergen exposure.

By considering the unique characteristics and needs of each patient, as well as the appropriate application techniques and monitoring for potential side effects, healthcare providers can ensure the optimal use of topical treatments and maximize the benefits for individuals with contact dermatitis.

As you continue your journey through this comprehensive guide, the next chapter will delve into the various systemic (oral and injectable) treatment options available for the management of contact dermatitis, equipping you with a thorough understanding of when and how to incorporate these therapies into the overall treatment plan.

CHAPTER 11

C hapter 11: Systemic Treatments for Contact Dermatitis

While topical therapies play a central role in the management of contact dermatitis, there are certain situations where systemic (oral or injectable) treatments may be necessary to effectively address the condition. These broader, whole-body approaches can provide an additional level of control over the inflammatory response and help alleviate symptoms that may not be adequately managed with localized topical treatments alone.

In this chapter, we will explore the various systemic treatment options available for contact dermatitis, including oral antihistamines, oral corticosteroids, and immunosuppressant drugs. We will delve into the mechanisms of action, appropriate indications, and potential side effects of each therapy, empowering both patients and healthcare providers to make informed decisions and develop comprehensive, evidence-based management strategies.

By understanding the strengths and limitations of systemic treatments for contact dermatitis, you will be better equipped to work collaboratively with your healthcare team to determine the most suitable approach for your specific needs and ensure the best possible outcomes.

Oral Antihistamines

Oral antihistamines are a commonly used systemic therapy in the management of allergic contact dermatitis (ACD), as they can help alleviate the characteristic symptoms associated with the condition.

Mechanism of Action

Antihistamines work by blocking the effects of histamine, a key mediator of the allergic inflammatory response. Histamine is released by mast cells and other immune cells when the skin encounters an allergen, triggering the symptoms of ACD, such as itching, redness, and swelling.

By inhibiting the binding of histamine to its receptors, oral antihistamines can help reduce the intensity of these allergic symptoms and provide relief for the patient.

Types of Oral Antihistamines

There are two main classes of oral antihistamines used in the management of ACD:

1. First-Generation Antihistamines:
   - Examples: Diphenhydramine, chlorpheniramine, dexchlorpheniramine
   - These older-generation antihistamines tend to have a more potent antipruritic (anti-itching) effect, making them useful for managing the intense itching associated with ACD.
   - However, they also have a higher risk of causing sedation and other central nervous system (CNS) side effects.

2. Second-Generation Antihistamines:
   - Examples: Cetirizine, loratadine, fexofenadine
   - These newer-generation antihistamines are generally less sedating and have a more favorable side effect profile compared to the first-generation options.
   - While they may be slightly less effective at relieving itching, they can provide a good balance of symptom control and tolerability.

Healthcare providers will typically consider factors such as the severity of the patient's symptoms, the potential for sedation, and the individual's response to determine the most appropriate oral antihistamine for the management of ACD.

Indications and Usage

Oral antihistamines are primarily indicated for the management of the acute, symptomatic phase of allergic contact dermatitis. They can be particularly useful in the following situations:

- Providing relief from intense itching and other allergic symptoms
    - Addressing flare-ups or exacerbations of ACD, especially when topical treatments alone are not sufficient
    - Complementing the use of topical therapies, such as corticosteroids or calcineurin inhibitors, to provide more comprehensive symptom control

Healthcare providers may recommend the use of oral antihistamines on a short-term, as-needed basis or as part of a more long-term management strategy, depending on the patient's individual needs and the severity of their condition.

Potential Side Effects

While oral antihistamines are generally well-tolerated, they can be associated with several potential side effects, including:

- Sedation and drowsiness (more common with first-generation antihistamines)
    - Dry mouth, blurred vision, and urinary retention
    - Dizziness, headache, and gastrointestinal disturbances

Patients should be advised to exercise caution when engaging in activities that require alertness or coordination, particularly during the initial stages of treatment or when using first-generation antihistamines.

Oral Corticosteroids

In cases of severe or widespread contact dermatitis, where topical treatments and oral antihistamines are not sufficient, healthcare providers may recommend the use of oral corticosteroids to rapidly reduce the skin's inflammatory response and provide relief.

Mechanism of Action
Oral corticosteroids, such as prednisone or methylprednisolone, work by inhibiting the production and activity of various inflammatory mediators, including cytokines, prostaglandins, and leukotrienes. This broad-spectrum anti-inflammatory effect can help alleviate the symptoms of both irritant and allergic contact dermatitis.

Indications and Usage
Oral corticosteroids are typically reserved for the management of acute, severe, or recalcitrant cases of contact dermatitis, where the skin condition is significantly impacting the patient's quality of life or ability to function. Some common indications for the use of oral corticosteroids include:

- Widespread, severe, or extensive contact dermatitis that is not responding adequately to topical treatments
  - Acute flare-ups or exacerbations of the condition that require rapid control of symptoms
  - Situations where the patient's occupation or daily activities are significantly impaired due to the severity of the skin condition

Healthcare providers will often prescribe a short course of oral corticosteroids, typically ranging from 5 to 14 days, to achieve rapid control of the inflammatory response. Patients may then be transitioned to topical or other systemic therapies to maintain long-term management of the condition.

Dosing and Tapering

The appropriate dosage of oral corticosteroids for the management of contact dermatitis will depend on the severity of the condition, the patient's body weight, and the healthcare provider's clinical judgment. Typical starting doses may range from 0.5 to 1 mg/kg of body weight per day, with the dose gradually tapered over the course of the treatment period.

Careful tapering of the oral corticosteroid dose is crucial to avoid the potential for withdrawal symptoms, such as joint pain, fatigue, and the rebound exacerbation of the skin condition. Healthcare providers will typically provide a detailed tapering schedule to ensure a smooth and safe transition off the systemic medication.

Potential Side Effects

Oral corticosteroids are associated with a range of potential side effects, particularly with prolonged use or high-dose therapy. Some of the most common side effects include:

- Weight gain, fluid retention, and the development of "moon face"
    - Increased risk of infection due to immunosuppression
    - Gastrointestinal disturbances, such as peptic ulcers or heartburn
    - Metabolic changes, including hyperglycemia and electrolyte imbalances
    - Mood changes, insomnia, and other neuropsychiatric effects

Healthcare providers must carefully weigh the risks and benefits of using oral corticosteroids, particularly in patients with pre-existing medical conditions or those who require long-term management of their contact dermatitis.

Immunosuppressant Drugs

In rare, severe, or treatment-resistant cases of contact dermatitis, healthcare providers may consider the use of systemic immunosuppressant medications to help control the underlying inflammatory and immune-mediated processes.

Mechanism of Action

Immunosuppressant drugs, such as cyclosporine, methotrexate, and mycophenolate mofetil, work by targeting specific components of the immune system that are responsible for the development and perpetuation of the allergic or inflammatory response in contact dermatitis.

By disrupting the signaling pathways and inhibiting the activity of key immune cells, these medications can help reduce the intensity of the skin's reaction and provide more comprehensive control of the condition.

Indications and Usage

Systemic immunosuppressant drugs are typically reserved for the management of severe, chronic, or treatment-resistant cases of contact dermatitis, where other therapies, including topical treatments and oral corticosteroids, have been ineffective or are not feasible for long-term use. Some common indications for the use of immunosuppressant drugs in the context of contact dermatitis include:

- Severe, widespread, or disabling cases of allergic contact dermatitis that are not responding to other treatments
  - Chronic, recurrent forms of irritant or allergic contact dermatitis that significantly impact the patient's quality of life and daily functioning
  - Situations where the prolonged use of topical or oral corticosteroids is contraindicated or not well-tolerated

Healthcare providers will carefully evaluate the risks and benefits of using immunosuppressant drugs, taking into consideration the patient's overall health status, the severity of the skin condition, and the potential for adverse effects.

Specific Immunosuppressant Drugs

1. Cyclosporine:

- A potent immunosuppressant that inhibits the activation and proliferation of T cells, a key component of the allergic response.

- Typically used for short-term management of severe or recalcitrant contact dermatitis, with close monitoring for potential side effects, such as kidney or liver dysfunction.

2. Methotrexate:

- An antimetabolite drug that disrupts the division and proliferation of rapidly dividing cells, including activated immune cells.

- May be considered for the long-term management of chronic, recurrent contact dermatitis, with careful monitoring for potential side effects, such as bone marrow suppression or liver toxicity.

3. Mycophenolate mofetil:

- An immunosuppressant that inhibits the proliferation of lymphocytes, a type of immune cell involved in the allergic response.

- Can be used as a steroid-sparing agent in the management of chronic, treatment-resistant contact dermatitis, with close monitoring for potential gastrointestinal or infectious complications.

Potential Side Effects
Systemic immunosuppressant drugs are associated with a range of potential side effects, which can vary depending on the specific medication and the duration of use. Some common side effects include:

- Increased susceptibility to infections, due to the overall suppression of the immune system
    - Gastrointestinal disturbances, such as nausea, vomiting, or diarrhea
    - Kidney or liver dysfunction, requiring regular monitoring and dose adjustments
    - Bone marrow suppression, leading to changes in blood cell counts
    - Neurological effects, such as headaches, dizziness, or fatigue

Healthcare providers must carefully weigh the risks and benefits of using systemic immunosuppressant drugs, closely monitor the patient's response and safety parameters, and provide comprehensive patient education to ensure the best possible outcomes.

Integrating Systemic Treatments into the Management Plan

When considering the use of systemic treatments for contact dermatitis, healthcare providers must carefully integrate these therapies into the overall management plan, taking into account the patient's individual needs, the severity of the condition, and the potential for synergistic effects with topical treatments.

Comprehensive Assessment
Before initiating any systemic therapy, healthcare providers should conduct a thorough assessment of the patient's medical history, current symptoms, and response to previous treatments. This evaluation can help guide the selection of the most appropriate systemic medication and determine the appropriate dosage and duration of treatment.

Coordination with Topical Therapies
In many cases, systemic treatments for contact dermatitis are used in conjunction with topical therapies, such as corticosteroids or calcineurin inhibitors. Healthcare providers must carefully coordinate the use of these various treatments to ensure they are compatible, effectively address the underlying condition, and do not result in any adverse interactions or compounding side effects.

Monitoring and Adjustments
Patients receiving systemic treatments for contact dermatitis require close monitoring and follow-up care to assess the effectiveness of the therapy, monitor for any adverse effects, and make necessary adjustments to the management plan. This may involve regular check-ins, laboratory testing,

and the careful titration of medication doses based on the patient's response and tolerability.

Patient Education and Adherence

Effective management of contact dermatitis with systemic treatments requires active engagement and adherence from the patient. Healthcare providers should provide comprehensive education on the rationale for the selected therapy, the expected timeline for improvement, and the importance of adhering to the prescribed regimen. Encouraging open communication and addressing any concerns or questions can help improve the patient's understanding and commitment to the treatment plan.

By taking a comprehensive, collaborative approach to the integration of systemic treatments into the management of contact dermatitis, healthcare providers can optimize the effectiveness of these therapies and ensure the best possible outcomes for their patients.

Conclusion

In this chapter, we have explored the role of systemic treatments in the management of contact dermatitis, including the use of oral antihistamines, oral corticosteroids, and immunosuppressant drugs.

Oral antihistamines can be a valuable adjunct to topical therapies, particularly in the management of allergic contact dermatitis, as they can help alleviate the characteristic symptoms, such as intense itching and swelling. Oral corticosteroids, on the other hand, may be necessary for the rapid control of severe or widespread cases of contact dermatitis that are not responding adequately to other treatments.

In rare, recalcitrant cases, healthcare providers may consider the use of systemic immunosuppressant medications, such as cyclosporine, methotrexate, or mycophenolate mofetil, to help control the underlying inflammatory and immune-mediated processes driving the skin condition. However, the use of these powerful drugs requires careful consideration of the risks and benefits, as well as close monitoring to ensure the best possible outcomes.

Integrating systemic treatments into the overall management plan for contact dermatitis involves a comprehensive assessment of the patient's needs, coordination with topical therapies, and ongoing monitoring and adjustments to the treatment regimen. Effective patient education and adherence are also crucial to the success of these broader, whole-body approaches to managing this complex skin condition.

As you continue your journey through this comprehensive guide, the next chapter will focus on the lifestyle and home management strategies that can complement the medical treatments and empower patients to take a more active role in the long-term management of their contact dermatitis.

CHAPTER 12

Chapter 12: Lifestyle and Home Management

While medical treatments, whether topical or systemic, are essential in the management of contact dermatitis, the role of lifestyle and home-based strategies should not be overlooked. These complementary approaches can play a crucial part in supporting the overall treatment plan, minimizing the risk of flare-ups, and promoting long-term skin health and well-being.

In this chapter, we will explore a range of lifestyle and home management strategies that can be implemented by individuals with contact dermatitis. From developing effective skin care routines to avoiding triggers within the home environment, and incorporating stress management techniques, we will provide comprehensive guidance to help patients take a proactive role in the management of their condition.

By understanding the importance of these holistic approaches and how to effectively integrate them into their daily lives, individuals with contact dermatitis can work in collaboration with their healthcare providers to achieve the best possible outcomes and maintain optimal skin health.

Skin Care Routines

Establishing and maintaining a gentle, consistent skin care routine is a crucial component of managing contact dermatitis, as it can help strengthen the skin's barrier function, reduce irritation, and prevent future flare-ups.

Cleansing

When it comes to cleansing the skin, individuals with contact dermatitis should opt for fragrance-free, pH-balanced, and hypoallergenic products. Harsh soaps, detergents, and cleansers can strip the skin of its natural oils and compromise the skin barrier, exacerbating the symptoms of contact dermatitis.

Gentle, creamy cleansers or non-soap-based cleansers are often the best choice, as they can effectively remove dirt and impurities without disrupting the skin's delicate balance. Patients should also be mindful of the frequency of cleansing, as over-washing can further irritate the skin.

Moisturizing

Proper moisturization is essential for individuals with contact dermatitis, as it helps to hydrate the skin, restore the skin barrier, and prevent further irritation or allergen exposure.

When selecting moisturizers, patients should opt for fragrance-free, hypoallergenic, and, ideally, fragrance-free formulations that are rich in emollient ingredients, such as petrolatum, ceramides, and glycerin. These types of moisturizers can help replenish the skin's natural lipids and strengthen the stratum corneum, which is often compromised in contact dermatitis.

Patients should be encouraged to apply moisturizers immediately after bathing or cleansing, when the skin is still damp, to lock in hydration and prevent evaporation.

Sun Protection

Sun exposure can exacerbate certain types of contact dermatitis, particularly in individuals with photosensitive reactions or photo-irritant contact dermatitis. Therefore, incorporating sun protection into the daily skin care routine is essential.

Patients should use broad-spectrum, fragrance-free sunscreens with a minimum Sun Protection Factor (SPF) of 30, and reapply the product regularly, especially when spending extended periods outdoors. In addition to sunscreen, the use of protective clothing, hats, and seeking shade can further minimize the risk of sun-induced flare-ups.

Bathing and Showering
The way individuals with contact dermatitis approach bathing and showering can also have a significant impact on their skin health. Patients should be advised to:

- Use lukewarm water, as hot water can strip the skin of its natural oils and lead to further irritation.
- Limit the duration of bathing or showering to 5-10 minutes to avoid prolonged exposure to water.
- Avoid scrubbing or using rough washcloths, which can further compromise the skin barrier.
- Gently pat the skin dry after bathing, rather than vigorously rubbing.

By incorporating these gentle skin care practices into their daily routine, individuals with contact dermatitis can help maintain the skin's protective function and minimize the risk of flare-ups.

Avoiding Triggers in the Home

The home environment can be a significant source of potential irritants and allergens that can trigger or exacerbate contact dermatitis. Identifying and eliminating these triggers within the home setting is a crucial aspect of the overall management strategy.

Household Cleaning Products

Many common household cleaning products, such as detergents, disin-fectants, and degreasers, can contain a variety of chemicals and fragrances that can act as skin irritants or allergens. Patients should be encouraged to replace these products with fragrance-free, hypoallergenic alternatives, or consider using natural, plant-based cleaning solutions.

Textiles and Fabrics

The materials used in clothing, bedding, and other household textiles can also contribute to contact dermatitis. Patients should opt for natural, breathable fabrics, such as cotton or linen, and avoid synthetic materials, wool, and fabrics with chemical finishes or dyes.

Washing all household textiles with fragrance-free, hypoallergenic detergents can also help minimize the risk of exposure to potential triggers.

Personal Care Products

Similar to household cleaning products, many personal care items, such as soaps, shampoos, lotions, and cosmetics, can contain fragrances, preser-vatives, and other ingredients that may trigger contact dermatitis. Patients should carefully read labels and choose fragrance-free, hypoallergenic alternatives for all personal care products used within the home.

Pest Control and Landscaping

Exposure to certain plants, insects, or chemicals used for pest control or landscaping can also lead to the development of contact dermatitis. Patients should be mindful of any outdoor activities or landscaping work that may involve potential triggers, such as poisonous plants or insecticides, and take appropriate precautions.

Indoor Air Quality

The air quality within the home can also impact individuals with contact dermatitis. Factors such as dust, mold, and volatile organic compounds

(VOCs) from household products or furnishings can contribute to skin irritation. Patients should consider using air purifiers, maintaining proper ventilation, and avoiding the use of scented candles or air fresheners.

By carefully assessing and addressing the potential triggers within the home environment, patients can take an active role in minimizing the risk of contact dermatitis flare-ups and promoting overall skin health.

Stress Management Techniques

Stress and psychological factors can play a significant role in the development and exacerbation of contact dermatitis, as they can influence the skin's inflammatory response and immune function. Incorporating effective stress management techniques into the overall management plan can be a valuable complement to medical treatments.

Understanding the Link Between Stress and Skin Health

Chronic stress can lead to the activation of the body's stress response systems, resulting in the release of various inflammatory mediators, such as cytokines and neuropeptides. These substances can directly impact the skin, contributing to increased inflammation, impaired barrier function, and a heightened sensitivity to irritants or allergens.

Additionally, stress can also influence behavioral factors, such as increased scratching or picking of the skin, which can further exacerbate the symptoms of contact dermatitis.

Relaxation Techniques

Incorporating relaxation techniques into daily routines can help individuals with contact dermatitis manage stress and its associated effects on the skin. Some effective options include:

1. Meditation and mindfulness practices: Techniques such as deep breathing,

progressive muscle relaxation, and guided imagery can help calm the mind and reduce stress levels.

2. Yoga and gentle exercise: Low-impact physical activities can promote relaxation, improve mood, and reduce stress-induced inflammation.

3. Biofeedback and relaxation therapies: These techniques, which involve the use of specialized equipment to monitor and control physiological processes, can help patients learn to better manage their stress responses.

4. Massage and acupuncture: These complementary therapies can help alleviate muscle tension, improve circulation, and promote overall relaxation.

By regularly practicing these stress management techniques, patients can help mitigate the impact of psychological factors on their skin health and potentially reduce the frequency and severity of contact dermatitis flare-ups.

Emotional Support and Counseling

The emotional and psychosocial impact of living with a chronic skin condition like contact dermatitis can be significant, leading to feelings of frustration, anxiety, and depression. Providing patients with access to emotional support and counseling can be a valuable component of the overall management strategy.

Healthcare providers can recommend support groups, online forums, or individual therapy sessions with mental health professionals to help patients cope with the challenges of living with contact dermatitis. By addressing the emotional and psychological aspects of the condition, patients can develop healthier coping mechanisms and improve their overall quality of life.

Incorporating Lifestyle Changes

In addition to establishing effective skin care routines, avoiding triggers within the home, and incorporating stress management techniques, patients with contact dermatitis may also benefit from making broader lifestyle changes to support their overall skin health and well-being.

Dietary Modifications

While there is limited evidence that specific dietary factors directly cause or exacerbate contact dermatitis, some patients may find that certain foods or food additives can trigger or worsen their skin condition. Patients should be encouraged to pay attention to any potential food-related triggers and consider the following dietary modifications:

- Eliminating or reducing the consumption of known food allergens, such as certain fruits, vegetables, or preservatives.
- Incorporating a balanced, nutrient-rich diet that supports skin health, including foods rich in antioxidants, healthy fats, and vitamins.
- Staying hydrated by drinking an adequate amount of water throughout the day.

Healthcare providers may also recommend working with a registered dietitian or nutritionist to develop a personalized dietary plan that supports the management of contact dermatitis.

Exercise and Physical Activity

Regular physical activity can have a positive impact on the management of contact dermatitis by:

- Reducing stress and promoting overall well-being, which can help mitigate the impact of psychological factors on the skin.
- Improving circulation and lymphatic drainage, which can support the skin's natural healing processes.
- Maintaining a healthy weight, as excess weight can exacerbate certain types of contact dermatitis, such as intertriginous or inverse dermatitis.

Patients should be encouraged to engage in gentle, low-impact exercises that do not further irritate the skin, such as walking, swimming, or low-intensity yoga.

Lifestyle Adjustments in the Workplace

For individuals with occupational contact dermatitis, making certain adjustments in the workplace can be crucial for managing their condition and preventing future flare-ups. These adjustments may include:

- Collaborating with employers to implement engineering controls, such as improved ventilation or containment systems, to minimize exposure to potential triggers.
- Utilizing personal protective equipment (PPE), such as gloves or protective clothing, to create a barrier between the skin and potential irritants or allergens.
- Exploring the possibility of job modifications or reassignment to reduce exposure to known triggers within the work environment.

By incorporating these comprehensive lifestyle and home management strategies into the overall treatment plan, patients with contact dermatitis can take a more proactive and holistic approach to managing their condition, promoting long-term skin health, and improving their overall quality of life.

Ongoing Monitoring and Adjustment

Effective management of contact dermatitis requires a continuous process of monitoring, evaluation, and adjustment of the patient's lifestyle and home-based strategies. Maintaining open communication with healthcare providers and being willing to adapt to changing needs is crucial for the long-term success of these complementary approaches.

Regular Check-ins and Assessments

Patients should be encouraged to schedule regular check-ins with their healthcare providers, either in person or through virtual visits, to discuss the efficacy of their lifestyle and home management strategies. During these appointments, the healthcare provider can:

- Evaluate the patient's skin condition and monitor for any changes or new developments.
    - Assess the patient's adherence to the recommended skin care routines, avoidance of triggers, and stress management techniques.
    - Provide guidance on adjusting or refining the home management strategies based on the patient's evolving needs and the healthcare provider's clinical assessment.

This ongoing dialogue and collaborative approach can help ensure that the home-based management strategies remain effective and aligned with the patient's overall treatment plan.

Adapting to Changes and Challenges
Contact dermatitis can be a dynamic and, at times, unpredictable condition, with changes in triggers, symptoms, and the patient's overall health and lifestyle. Patients must be prepared to adapt their home management strategies as needed to address these fluctuations.

For example, if a patient identifies a new trigger within their home environment or experiences a significant life event that increases their stress levels, they may need to re-evaluate and modify their approach to avoid future flare-ups. By maintaining flexibility and a willingness to make adjustments, patients can ensure the continued effectiveness of their home-based management strategies.

Collaboration with Healthcare Providers
The success of the home management strategies for contact dermatitis often relies on the patient's ability to work collaboratively with their healthcare providers. This includes:

- Keeping detailed records or logs of skin condition, trigger exposures, and the effectiveness of various home-based interventions.

- Communicating openly and honestly with healthcare providers about any challenges, concerns, or new developments related to the patient's condition.

- Actively participating in the decision-making process and being receptive to the healthcare provider's recommendations for adjusting the home management plan.

By fostering this collaborative partnership, patients and healthcare providers can continuously optimize the home-based management strategies and ensure the best possible outcomes in the long-term management of contact dermatitis.

Conclusion

In this chapter, we have explored the crucial role of lifestyle and home management strategies in the comprehensive approach to managing contact dermatitis. From establishing gentle skin care routines and avoiding triggers within the home environment to incorporating stress management techniques and making broader lifestyle adjustments, these complementary approaches can significantly contribute to the overall success of the treatment plan.

By empowering patients to take a proactive role in the management of their condition, these home-based strategies can help improve skin health, reduce the frequency and severity of flare-ups, and enhance the patient's overall quality of life. Importantly, we have emphasized the need for ongoing monitoring, evaluation, and adaptation of these strategies to ensure they remain effective and aligned with the patient's evolving needs.

Ultimately, the successful management of contact dermatitis requires a collaborative effort between patients and healthcare providers, with both parties working together to integrate the medical treatments and the lifestyle and home-based interventions. By adopting this comprehensive, holistic approach, individuals with contact dermatitis can achieve the best possible outcomes and take control of their skin health.

As you continue your journey through this guide, the next chapter will explore the role of complementary and alternative therapies in the management of contact dermatitis, providing an overview of botanical remedies, dietary modifications, and mind-body practices that may serve as valuable adjuncts to the overall treatment plan.

CHAPTER 13

C hapter 13: Complementary and Alternative Therapies

While conventional medical treatments, including topical and systemic therapies, remain the foundation of contact dermatitis management, there is growing interest and utilization of complementary and alternative therapies (CAT) as adjuncts to the overall treatment plan. These holistic approaches can offer additional benefits, such as reducing symptoms, modulating the underlying inflammatory processes, and promoting overall skin health and well-being.

In this chapter, we will explore several complementary and alternative therapies that may be beneficial for individuals with contact dermatitis. We will discuss the potential mechanisms of action, the available scientific evidence, and the appropriate integration of these modalities into the comprehensive management strategy. By understanding the potential role and limitations of CAT, patients and healthcare providers can make informed decisions and work collaboratively to determine the most suitable approach for each individual's needs.

Botanical Remedies

The use of botanical remedies, or herbal medicines, has a long-standing tradition in the treatment of various skin conditions, including contact dermatitis. While the scientific evidence is still emerging, several plant-based compounds have shown promise in the management of this skin condition.

Topical Botanical Treatments

Certain botanical extracts can be formulated into topical preparations, such as creams, ointments, or lotions, and applied directly to the affected skin. Some of the more commonly studied topical botanical treatments for contact dermatitis include:

1. Calendula (Calendula officinalis):
   - Calendula has demonstrated anti-inflammatory, antimicrobial, and wound-healing properties that may be beneficial in the management of contact dermatitis.
   - Topical preparations containing calendula extract have been used to soothe and promote the healing of skin lesions associated with contact dermatitis.

2. Chamomile (Matricaria recutita):
   - Chamomile is known for its anti-inflammatory, antioxidant, and skin-soothing properties, which may help alleviate the symptoms of contact dermatitis.
   - Topical chamomile preparations have been used to reduce redness, itching, and skin irritation in individuals with contact dermatitis.

3. Aloe vera (Aloe barbadensis):
   - Aloe vera is widely recognized for its wound-healing, anti-inflammatory, and moisturizing properties, which can be beneficial in the management of contact dermatitis.
   - Topical aloe vera gel or ointments may help soothe the skin and promote healing during flare-ups.

It is essential to note that while these botanical remedies have shown promise, the quality, safety, and efficacy of topical botanical products can vary significantly. Patients should consult with their healthcare providers before using any topical botanical treatments, as they may interact with conventional medications or exacerbate certain skin conditions.

Oral Botanical Supplements

In addition to topical applications, some botanical remedies can be taken orally in the form of supplements or teas. These botanical supplements may have the potential to modulate the underlying inflammatory processes associated with contact dermatitis. Examples of oral botanical supplements that have been studied for their potential benefits include:

1. Quercetin:
   - Quercetin is a flavonoid compound found in various plants that has demonstrated anti-inflammatory and antioxidant properties.
   - Some studies suggest that oral quercetin supplementation may help reduce the severity of allergic contact dermatitis by modulating the immune response.

2. Omega-3 fatty acids:
   - Omega-3 fatty acids, such as those found in fish oil or flaxseed, have been shown to possess anti-inflammatory effects that may be beneficial in the management of contact dermatitis.
   - Oral supplementation with omega-3 fatty acids may help reduce the severity of symptoms and prevent flare-ups.

3. Curcumin:
   - Curcumin, the active compound in turmeric, has been studied for its anti-inflammatory, antioxidant, and skin-protective properties.
   - Some research suggests that oral curcumin supplementation may help alleviate the symptoms of contact dermatitis and improve the overall skin condition.

As with topical botanical treatments, it is essential for patients to consult with their healthcare providers before starting any oral botanical supplements, as they may interact with conventional medications or have potential side effects, especially in individuals with underlying medical conditions.

Dietary Modifications

While there is limited evidence that specific dietary factors directly cause or exacerbate contact dermatitis, some patients may find that certain foods or dietary patterns can trigger or worsen their skin condition. Incorporating dietary modifications as part of the overall management strategy may, therefore, be a valuable complement to conventional treatments.

Elimination Diets
Some individuals with contact dermatitis may benefit from following an elimination diet, which involves temporarily removing specific foods or food groups from the diet to identify potential triggers. Common food allergens that have been associated with contact dermatitis include:

- Nuts and seeds
    - Certain fruits and vegetables
    - Dairy products
    - Wheat and gluten-containing grains

By systematically eliminating and then reintroducing these foods, patients can determine if their skin condition is influenced by specific dietary factors and make appropriate adjustments to their long-term dietary habits.

Anti-Inflammatory Diets
In addition to identifying and avoiding potential trigger foods, adopting an anti-inflammatory dietary pattern may also be beneficial for individuals with contact dermatitis. An anti-inflammatory diet typically emphasizes the consumption of:

- Whole, unprocessed foods

- Fruits and vegetables rich in antioxidants
- Healthy fats, such as those found in fatty fish, nuts, and olive oil
- Probiotic-rich foods, like yogurt or fermented vegetables

The goal of an anti-inflammatory diet is to provide the body with a balanced intake of nutrients that can help modulate the underlying inflammatory processes associated with contact dermatitis and promote overall skin health.

Personalized Dietary Strategies

It is important to note that the impact of dietary factors on contact dermatitis can be highly individualized. What may trigger a reaction in one person may not affect another. Healthcare providers can work with patients to develop personalized dietary strategies that take into account the patient's specific symptoms, triggers, and overall health status.

By incorporating dietary modifications into the comprehensive management plan, patients with contact dermatitis may experience a reduction in symptoms, fewer flare-ups, and an improvement in their overall skin health and well-being.

Mind-Body Practices

As discussed in the previous chapter, stress and psychological factors can play a significant role in the development and exacerbation of contact dermatitis. Incorporating mind-body practices into the management strategy can, therefore, be a valuable complement to the conventional medical treatments and lifestyle interventions.

Meditation and Mindfulness

Practices that focus on cultivating present-moment awareness, such as meditation and mindfulness, can help individuals with contact dermatitis manage stress and promote relaxation. These techniques may work by:

- Reducing the production of stress hormones, such as cortisol, which can contribute to inflammation
- Modulating the immune system and inhibiting the release of pro-inflammatory cytokines
- Improving the ability to cope with the emotional and psychosocial aspects of living with a chronic skin condition

Regular practice of meditation and mindfulness can help individuals with contact dermatitis become more aware of their thought patterns, emotions, and bodily sensations, enabling them to respond to stressors in a more adaptive manner.

Yoga and Breathwork

Gentle yoga practices, which incorporate physical postures, breath control, and meditation, can also be beneficial for individuals with contact dermatitis. The combination of physical movement, breath awareness, and relaxation techniques can help:

- Reduce muscle tension and promote overall relaxation
- Improve circulation and lymphatic drainage, which can support the skin's healing processes
- Enhance the mind-body connection and foster a greater sense of well-being

Additionally, specific breathwork techniques, such as diaphragmatic breathing or pranayama, can help activate the parasympathetic nervous system, further promoting a state of calm and relaxation.

Biofeedback and Hypnotherapy

More specialized mind-body therapies, such as biofeedback and hypnotherapy, may also have a role in the management of contact dermatitis. These approaches involve the use of specialized equipment or techniques to:

- Provide real-time feedback on physiological processes, such as skin temperature or muscle tension, to help patients learn to better regulate their stress responses
  - Induce a state of deep relaxation and heightened suggestibility, which can be used to address the psychological and emotional aspects of the skin condition

While the scientific evidence for the use of these mind-body practices in the management of contact dermatitis is still emerging, they may serve as valuable adjuncts to conventional treatments, particularly for individuals who struggle with the emotional and psychosocial impact of their skin condition.

Integrating Complementary and Alternative Therapies

When considering the use of complementary and alternative therapies (CAT) in the management of contact dermatitis, it is essential to approach the integration of these modalities with a thoughtful and evidence-based approach. Patients and healthcare providers should work collaboratively to determine the most appropriate and safe way to incorporate CAT into the overall treatment plan.

Assessing the Evidence
  Before recommending or using any complementary or alternative therapy, it is important to carefully evaluate the available scientific evidence regarding its safety and efficacy in the context of contact dermatitis. Healthcare providers should review the latest research, consult with experts in the field, and consider the quality and strength of the available studies.

While some botanical remedies, dietary modifications, and mind-body practices have shown promise in preliminary research, the scientific evidence is still evolving, and the long-term effects and optimal dosing or application methods may not be fully established. Patients should be advised to approach the use of CAT with appropriate caution and in close consultation with their healthcare providers.

Addressing Safety Concerns
In addition to evaluating the evidence, healthcare providers must also consider the potential safety concerns associated with the use of complementary and alternative therapies. Factors to consider include:

- Potential interactions with conventional medications or other treatments
- Possible adverse effects or contraindications, especially in individuals with underlying medical conditions
- The quality, purity, and standardization of botanical or dietary supplements

Patients should be encouraged to disclose the use of any CAT to their healthcare providers, who can then assess the risks and benefits and provide guidance on the safe and appropriate integration of these modalities into the management plan.

Collaborative Decision-making
The decision to incorporate complementary and alternative therapies into the management of contact dermatitis should be a collaborative process between the patient and the healthcare provider. This involves:

1. Open communication: Patients should feel empowered to discuss their interest in and use of CAT with their healthcare providers, who should, in turn, be receptive to these conversations.

2. Shared decision-making: Healthcare providers and patients should work together to evaluate the available evidence, consider the individual's needs and preferences, and determine the most appropriate way to integrate CAT into the overall management strategy.

3. Ongoing monitoring and adjustment: The use of CAT should be regularly

reviewed, and the management plan should be adjusted as needed based on the patient's response and any new developments or safety concerns.

By adopting a collaborative, evidence-based approach to the integration of complementary and alternative therapies, patients and healthcare providers can optimize the benefits and minimize the potential risks associated with these holistic approaches to the management of contact dermatitis.

Conclusion

In this chapter, we have explored the role of complementary and alternative therapies (CAT) in the management of contact dermatitis, providing an overview of various botanical remedies, dietary modifications, and mind-body practices that may serve as valuable adjuncts to the conventional medical treatments.

While the scientific evidence for the use of CAT in the context of contact dermatitis is still emerging, several of these holistic approaches have shown promise in reducing symptoms, modulating the underlying inflammatory processes, and promoting overall skin health and well-being. These complementary therapies can be particularly beneficial for individuals who are interested in a more holistic approach to managing their skin condition.

It is essential, however, to approach the integration of CAT with appropriate caution and in close collaboration with healthcare providers. Patients should disclose the use of any complementary or alternative therapies, and healthcare providers should carefully evaluate the available evidence, assess the potential risks and benefits, and work with patients to determine the most suitable and safe way to incorporate these modalities into the overall management plan.

By adopting a comprehensive, evidence-based, and collaborative approach to the management of contact dermatitis, patients and healthcare providers can leverage the potential benefits of both conventional medical treatments and complementary and alternative therapies to achieve the best possible outcomes and promote long-term skin health and well-being.

As you continue your journey through this comprehensive guide, the final chapter will focus on the important aspects of living with and advocating for oneself in the context of contact dermatitis, empowering you with the knowledge and strategies to navigate the challenges of this chronic skin condition.

CHAPTER 14

Chapter 14: Living with Contact Dermatitis

Navigating the complexities of contact dermatitis can be a challenging and often isolating experience. Beyond the physical symptoms and the management of the condition, individuals living with contact dermatitis must also contend with the emotional, social, and practical implications of this chronic skin condition. Addressing these broader aspects of the patient experience is crucial for achieving optimal outcomes and maintaining a good quality of life.

In this final chapter, we will explore the emotional and psychosocial impacts of living with contact dermatitis, and provide strategies for coping, self-advocacy, and accessing the necessary resources and support networks. By empowering individuals with the knowledge and tools to navigate the complex landscape of contact dermatitis, this chapter aims to equip patients with the means to take control of their condition and advocate for their own well-being.

Coping with the Emotional Impacts

The physical symptoms and management challenges associated with contact dermatitis can have a significant impact on an individual's emotional and psychological well-being. Addressing these emotional aspects is an essential component of the comprehensive approach to managing this chronic skin condition.

Acknowledging the Emotional Burden
Living with a persistent, recurrent, and often visible skin condition like contact dermatitis can take a toll on an individual's mental health. Patients may experience a range of emotions, including:

- Frustration and Helplessness: The lack of a clear cure and the struggle to manage persistent symptoms can lead to feelings of frustration and a sense of helplessness.
  - Anxiety and Depression: The physical discomfort, social stigma, and disruption to daily activities can contribute to the development of anxiety and depression.
  - Low Self-Esteem and Body Image Issues: The appearance of the skin lesions and the social consequences can negatively impact an individual's self-esteem and body image.

Acknowledging the emotional burden of living with contact dermatitis is the first step in addressing these challenges and developing effective coping strategies.

Strategies for Emotional Coping
Healthcare providers can work with patients to implement various coping strategies and provide support to help mitigate the emotional impacts of contact dermatitis:

1. Counseling and Psychotherapy:
   - Referral to mental health professionals, such as therapists or psychologists, can provide patients with the tools and support to manage the emotional and psychological aspects of their condition.
   - Cognitive-behavioral therapy (CBT) and other evidence-based psychotherapeutic approaches can help patients develop healthier thought patterns, coping mechanisms, and stress management techniques.

2. Support Groups and Peer Connections:
   - Connecting with others who are living with contact dermatitis, either through in-person or online support groups, can help patients feel less isolated and provide a sense of community.
   - Sharing experiences, coping strategies, and practical tips with peers can be empowering and help patients feel understood and validated.

3. Relaxation and Stress Management:
   - Incorporating mind-body practices, such as meditation, yoga, or deep breathing exercises, can help patients manage stress and promote a sense of calm and well-being.
   - Engaging in regular physical activity, hobbies, or other enjoyable activities can also serve as an outlet for managing the emotional impacts of contact dermatitis.

4. Self-Care and Mindfulness:
   - Encouraging patients to prioritize self-care, such as engaging in relaxing skin care routines, can help them feel more in control of their condition and promote a sense of self-compassion.
   - Practicing mindfulness and being present in the moment can help patients navigate the ups and downs of living with a chronic skin condition.

By addressing the emotional and psychological aspects of contact dermatitis, healthcare providers can help patients develop a more comprehensive and resilient approach to managing their condition, ultimately improving their overall quality of life.

Advocating for Oneself

Effective self-advocacy is crucial for individuals living with contact dermatitis, as it empowers them to navigate the healthcare system, ensure their needs are met, and actively participate in the management of their condition.

Communicating with Healthcare Providers

Open and honest communication with healthcare providers is the foundation of effective self-advocacy. Patients should feel empowered to:

1. Express their concerns and priorities: Patients should be encouraged to share their symptoms, treatment preferences, and overall goals for managing their contact dermatitis.
2. Ask questions and seek clarification: Patients should not hesitate to ask for explanations about their condition, treatment options, and the rationale behind the recommended management plan.
3. Discuss any challenges or barriers to care: Patients should be proactive in discussing any obstacles they face, such as financial constraints, access to specialty care, or difficulty adhering to the prescribed regimen.

By fostering a collaborative partnership with healthcare providers, patients can ensure that the management of their contact dermatitis is tailored to their individual needs and preferences.

Navigating the Healthcare System

Successfully navigating the healthcare system can be a daunting task for individuals with contact dermatitis, particularly when it comes to accessing appropriate care, obtaining necessary medical supplies, or securing insurance coverage.

Patients should be empowered to:

1. Research their rights and entitlements: Patients should familiarize themselves with their healthcare coverage, worker's compensation benefits (if applicable), and any local or national resources that may be available to support their management of contact dermatitis.

2. Advocate for necessary accommodations: Patients should be prepared to advocate for reasonable accommodations in the workplace, school, or other settings to mitigate the impact of their condition on their daily activities.
3. Seek assistance from patient advocates or navigators: Connecting with patient advocacy organizations or healthcare system navigators can help patients overcome barriers to accessing the care and resources they need.

By taking an active role in navigating the healthcare system, patients can ensure that they receive the comprehensive and personalized care required to manage their contact dermatitis effectively.

Educating Others

In addition to advocating for themselves within the healthcare system, patients with contact dermatitis may also find it necessary to educate others about their condition, particularly in social or professional settings.

Patients should be empowered to:

1. Provide clear explanations about contact dermatitis: Patients should be prepared to explain the nature of their condition, including the triggers, symptoms, and management strategies, to help reduce misconceptions and foster understanding.
2. Advocate for workplace accommodations: In the workplace, patients should be willing to educate employers and colleagues about their condition and the need for reasonable accommodations, such as modified work duties or the use of protective equipment.
3. Raise awareness and combat stigma: By sharing their experiences and educating others, patients can help reduce the social stigma associated with contact dermatitis and create a more supportive and understanding

environment.

By taking an active role in educating others, patients can not only improve their own quality of life but also contribute to the broader awareness and understanding of contact dermatitis within their communities.

Resources and Support Networks

Living with contact dermatitis can be a challenging and isolating experience, but patients do not have to navigate this journey alone. There are a variety of resources and support networks available to help individuals with contact dermatitis manage their condition and maintain their overall well-being.

Patient Advocacy Organizations

Patient advocacy organizations dedicated to skin health and dermatological conditions can be invaluable sources of information, support, and resources for individuals with contact dermatitis. These organizations may provide:

- Educational materials and resources about contact dermatitis
    - Peer support groups, both in-person and online
    - Guidance on navigating the healthcare system and accessing care
    - Advocacy efforts to raise awareness and address policy issues

Examples of such organizations include the National Eczema Association, the American Contact Dermatitis Society, and the International Federation of Psoriasis Associations, among others.

Online Communities and Forums

In the digital age, online communities and forums have become increasingly important for individuals with chronic skin conditions like contact dermatitis. These platforms provide patients with the opportunity to:

- Connect with others who share similar experiences
  - Exchange information, tips, and coping strategies
  - Find emotional support and a sense of community
  - Access educational resources and stay informed about the latest developments in contact dermatitis management

Popular online forums and social media groups dedicated to contact dermatitis and related skin conditions can be invaluable resources for patients.

Local and Regional Support Groups
In addition to national and online resources, patients with contact dermatitis may also benefit from participating in local or regional support groups. These in-person gatherings can provide a valuable opportunity for:

- Sharing experiences and coping strategies with others in the community
  - Receiving support and encouragement from peers facing similar challenges
  - Accessing information about local healthcare providers, resources, and support services
  - Engaging in group activities or educational sessions related to contact dermatitis management

Healthcare providers can often assist patients in identifying and connecting with local support group options.

Professional and Vocational Resources
For individuals with occupational contact dermatitis, accessing professional and vocational resources can be crucial for managing their condition and maintaining their employment.

These resources may include:

- Occupational health specialists and workplace accommodations programs

- Worker's compensation and disability benefits assistance
- Job training or transition support services
- Educational materials and guidance on workplace safety and exposure prevention

By connecting with these specialized resources, patients can navigate the complexities of occupational contact dermatitis and ensure that their needs are met in the workplace.

By taking advantage of the various resources and support networks available, individuals with contact dermatitis can feel empowered, informed, and supported in their journey to manage this chronic skin condition.

Conclusion

In this final chapter, we have explored the crucial aspects of living with and advocating for oneself in the context of contact dermatitis. Beyond the physical management of the condition, individuals with contact dermatitis must also contend with the emotional, social, and practical implications of this chronic skin disorder.

Addressing the emotional burden of contact dermatitis, including the development of effective coping strategies and the incorporation of mental health support, is an essential component of the comprehensive approach to managing this condition. Patients must also be empowered to advocate for themselves, communicate effectively with healthcare providers, and navigate the complexities of the healthcare system to ensure their needs are met.

Furthermore, we have emphasized the importance of accessing the various resources and support networks available to individuals with contact dermatitis, including patient advocacy organizations, online communities, local support groups, and specialized vocational resources. By connecting with these valuable sources of information, support, and guidance, patients can feel empowered, informed, and supported in their journey to manage this chronic skin condition.

As you reach the end of this comprehensive guide, it is our hope that you have gained a deeper understanding of the multifaceted nature of contact dermatitis and the holistic strategies required to achieve optimal skin health and well-being. By working collaboratively with healthcare providers and taking an active role in the management of your condition, you can navigate the challenges of contact dermatitis and maintain a good quality of life.

CONCLUSION

Throughout the pages of this comprehensive guide, we have explored the complex and multifaceted nature of contact dermatitis, delving into the underlying causes, diagnostic approaches, and evidence-based management strategies that healthcare providers and patients can employ to address this prevalent skin condition.

From the foundational understanding of the distinct types of contact dermatitis - irritant and allergic - to the specialized considerations for unique manifestations, such as hand, facial, and genital dermatitis, this book has aimed to provide readers with a thorough and well-rounded knowledge base. By addressing the epidemiology, risk factors, and diagnostic tools used to identify the specific triggers and allergens responsible for contact dermatitis, we have empowered both patients and healthcare providers to work collaboratively in uncovering the root causes of this skin condition.

Importantly, the management of contact dermatitis has been a central focus of this guide, with in-depth discussions on the diverse array of topical and systemic treatment options, as well as the crucial role of lifestyle and home-based strategies in promoting long-term skin health. Whether it's the use of corticosteroids, calcineurin inhibitors, or barrier creams and emollients, or the implementation of gentle skin care routines, trigger avoidance, and stress management techniques, readers have been equipped with the knowledge and tools necessary to develop personalized, evidence-based management plans.

Beyond the medical and lifestyle-based approaches, this book has also explored the potential benefits and appropriate integration of complementary and alternative therapies, acknowledging the growing interest and utilization of holistic modalities, such as botanical remedies, dietary modifications, and mind-body practices, as adjuncts to the overall management of contact dermatitis.

Importantly, the unique challenges and considerations surrounding occupational contact dermatitis have been addressed, recognizing the significant impact this skin condition can have on individuals' work lives, as well as the essential role of healthcare providers, employers, and regulatory authorities in collaboratively addressing this critical occupational health issue.

As readers progress through the final chapters of this guide, the focus shifts to the broader, yet equally crucial, aspects of living with and advocating for oneself in the context of contact dermatitis. By acknowledging the emotional and psychosocial impacts of this chronic skin condition and empowering individuals to effectively communicate with healthcare providers, navigate the healthcare system, and access the necessary resources and support networks, this book aims to provide a comprehensive, patient-centered approach to managing contact dermatitis.

Throughout this journey, the overarching goal has been to equip both patients and healthcare providers with the knowledge, strategies, and collaborative mindset required to achieve the best possible outcomes in the management of contact dermatitis. By fostering a deeper understanding of this complex skin condition and the multifaceted approaches to its prevention, diagnosis, and treatment, this guide serves as an invaluable resource for all those invested in the pursuit of optimal skin health and well-being.

As you reach the conclusion of this comprehensive exploration of contact dermatitis, it is our hope that you have gained a newfound appreciation for the far-reaching impact of this skin condition and the critical importance of continued research, education, and advocacy in this field. Whether you are a patient seeking to better understand and manage your own contact dermatitis, or a healthcare provider looking to enhance your clinical expertise, the knowledge and strategies presented within these pages can serve as a solid foundation for navigating the complexities of this prevalent and often-misunderstood skin condition.

As the landscape of contact dermatitis management continues to evolve, with emerging treatments, innovative diagnostic tools, and a deeper understanding of the underlying mechanisms, it is essential that patients, healthcare providers, and the broader community remain vigilant, adaptive, and committed to providing the highest quality of care and support. By fostering collaborative partnerships, embracing a holistic approach, and empowering individuals to take an active role in their own skin health, we can work collectively to minimize the burden of contact dermatitis and improve the overall quality of life for those affected by this challenging skin condition.